LOCAL ANESTHESIA FOR DERMATOLOGIC SURGERY

PRACTICAL MANUALS IN DERMATOLOGIC SURGERY

Series Consulting Editor
Roy C. Grekin, M.D.

Salasche/Grabski
FLAPS FOR THE CENTRAL FACE

Maloney
THE DERMATOLOGIC SURGICAL SUITE
Design and Materials

Skouge
SKIN GRAFTING

Zachary
BASIC CUTANEOUS SURGERY

Pollack
ELECTROSURGERY OF THE SKIN

Auletta/Grekin
LOCAL ANESTHESIA FOR DERMATOLOGIC
SURGERY

Forthcoming

Greenway/Breisch
CUTANEOUS SURGICAL ANATOMY OF THE
HEAD AND NECK

LOCAL ANESTHESIA FOR DERMATOLOGIC SURGERY

Michael J. Auletta, M.D.

Assistant Clinical Professor
Department of Medicine
University of Medicine and Dentistry of New Jersey
Robert Wood Johnson Medical School
Piscataway, New Jersey

Roy C. Grekin, M.D.

Associate Clinical Professor
Department of Dermatology
Chief of Dermatologic Surgery
University of California, San Francisco
School of Medicine
San Francisco, California

Illustrated by Kathleen Jee, B.F.A.

CHURCHILL LIVINGSTONE
New York, Edinburgh, London, Melbourne, Tokyo

Library of Congress Cataloging-in-Publication Data
Auletta, Michael J.
    Local anesthesia for dermatologic surgery / Michael J.
Auletta, Roy C. Grekin ; illustrated by Kathleen Jee.
      p. cm. — (Practical mauals in dermatologic surgery)
    Includes bibliographical references and index.
    ISBN 0-443-08704-0
    1. Local anesthesia. 2. Skin—Surgery. I. Grekin, Roy C.
II. Title. III. Series.
    [DNLM: 1. Anesthesia, Local. 2. Skin—surgery. WO 300 A924L]
    RD655.A85 1990
    DNLM/DLC
    for Library of Congress   90-15073
                                                CIP

© Churchill Livingstone Inc. 1991

Distributed in the United Kingdom by Churchill Livingstone, Robert Stevenson House, 1–3 Baxter's Place, Leith Walk, Edinburgh EH1 3AF, and by associated companies, branches, and representatives throughout the world.

Accurate indications, adverse reactions, and dosage schedules for drugs are provided in this book, but it is possible that they may change. The reader is urged to review the package information data of the manufacturers of the medications mentioned.

Acquisitions Editor: *Beth Kaufman Barry*
Copy Editor: *Marian Ryan*
Production Designer: *Charlie Lebeda*
Production Supervisor: *Jeanine Furino*

Printed in the United States of America

First published in 1991

To Mary and Edward Auletta

Michael Auletta

With love and appreciation to my parents, Bob and Shirley, for getting me to it, and to my family, Marta, Cortney, and Katie, for getting me through it

Roy Grekin

FOREWORD

As surgery becomes a more integral part of the practice of dermatology, it is necessary that the literature and training keep pace. Although surgical skills are currently being taught on a regular basis as part of the residency core curriculum, few "how to" manuals exist. Additionally, many practicing dermatologists wish to increase their surgical knowledge. The courses are available, but detailed instructional manuals for day to day office use are lacking.

In this spirit, this series, *Practical Manuals in Dermatologic Surgery,* was conceived. The manuals are designed to be "user friendly." Historical aspects and basic science information are excluded or mentioned only as absolutely necessary. The focus is purely on telling the reader how to perform specific procedures in a logical stepwise fashion.

Dermatologic surgery covers a wide gamut of areas; not all dermatologists wish to pursue every facet. Therefore, the series is divided into many small self-contained volumes to allow the clinician to purchase only those applicable to one's practice. As skills grow and new areas are approached additional titles can be added to form a complete library of surgical manuals.

The authors of each manual are noted experts within dermatologic surgery with a background in teaching. We are all very excited to participate in this new series as we are committed to dermatologic surgery and its role within our specialty. We hope you find these manuals of great practical use.

Roy C. Grekin, M.D.

PREFACE

Local anesthetics are truly remarkable drugs. Without these agents many of the advances in dermatologic surgery would not have been possible. Described as reversible regional loss of sensation, local anesthesia, delivered appropriately, can play an important role in allaying patient fears and in facilitating the surgical procedure.

Most physicians are familiar to some degree with the use of local anesthetics. However, there is much information on the subject that is not taught in residency programs nor found in standard dermatology or dermatologic surgery texts. Matching anesthetic duration to procedural length, various peripheral nerve blocks, and appropriate vasoconstrictor use can improve surgical efficiency. Buffered anesthetic solutions, variations in needle and syringe size, and other injection "tricks" can ease patient fears and discomfort. Knowledge of drug interactions, anesthetic toxicities, and treatments for adverse reactions can limit complications and minimize sequelae through early recognition and prompt appropriate response.

This practical manual is designed for "hands on" day to day application. We purposely de-emphasize history and basic science. The material is presented in an instructional stepwise fashion that "walks" the physician through each of the anesthetic procedures presented. While by no means a complete coverage of local anesthesia, this manual will provide both residents in training and practicing physicians with the expertise to deliver safe, thoughtful, and effective local anesthesia for most cutaneous surgical procedures.

Michael J. Auletta, M.D.
Roy C. Grekin, M.D.

CONTENTS

1

Mechanism of Anesthetic Action

Electric properties of nerve activity are based on the differential electrolyte concentrations between the extracellular fluid and the intracellular cytoplasm. They differ greatly. The extracellular fluid is high in sodium (Na^+) concentration and low in potassium (K^+) concentration. The opposite is true for the nerve cell cytoplasm. The resting cell membrane is poorly permeable to Na^+ ions, which allows maintenance of the Na^+ gradient across the membrane (Fig. 1-1).

When nerve excitation occurs, a rigid sequence of events is followed. Initially, a slow, gradual period of depolarization occurs as a result of Na^+ ion influx across the nerve cell membrane. When the transmembrane electric potential decreases from its resting potential (approximately -70 mV) to between -60 and -50 mV, a threshold or firing potential is achieved. At that point, Na^+ ion permeability across the membrane greatly increases, thereby allowing a rapid Na^+ ion influx and associated depolarization to approximately $+40$ mV.

When depolarization is complete the permeability of the nerve cell membrane changes, becoming once again relatively impermeable to Na^+ ions. The -70 mV resting potential is initially reached because of the outflow of K^+ ions. Once the resting potential is achieved, the excess of Na^+ ions within the cell and K^+ ions outside the cell is reversed by action of an ATP-driven Na^+–K^+ pump which restores the electrophysiologic status of the nerve to its normal resting state.

Studies have shown that the primary action of local anesthetics is inhibiting the depolarization phase of the excitation process. This is achieved by interfering with the influx of Na^+ ions, which prevents the action potential from reaching the firing (threshold) level and therefore blocks propagation of the electric impulse along the nerve.

The exact mechanism by which local anesthetics block the Na^+ ion movement across the nerve cell membrane is not known, but two theories have been proposed. The first is the *specific receptor theory*. In this proposed

1

TRANSMEMBRANE ACTION POTENTIAL

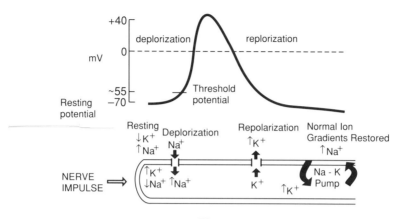

Figure 1-1

mechanism of action, the local anesthetic diffuses across the cell membrane to the internal surface and binds to a specific receptor at the opening of the sodium channel. This action alters either the structure or the function of the channel, thereby inhibiting Na^+ ion movement. The second proposed mechanism of action is offered by the *membrane expansion theory*. In this theory the local anesthetic is nonspecifically absorbed within the cell membrane. This results in an expansion of the membrane and subsequent narrowing of the sodium channels. It is possible that both mechanisms play a role in anesthetic action.

STRUCTURE-ACTIVITY FUNCTIONS

Pharmacokinetic activities of local anesthetics depend on their abilities to both diffuse across the nerve cell membrane and to bind to intracellular receptors. Agents that are more highly lipid soluble diffuse more readily and efficiently across cell membranes and therefore produce more potent anesthesia (i.e., lower concentrations needed). However, duration of activity is a function of protein binding. Anesthetics with a higher degree of protein (receptor) binding produce a longer period of action (Table 1-1).

The basic anesthetic structure consists of an aromatic group at one end and an amine group at the other, which are connected by an intermediate hydrocarbon chain (Fig. 1-2).

Whereas the aromatic moiety is primarily responsible for the lipophilic nature of these agents, changes in either the aromatic or amine group can alter lipid/water solubility characteristics. Again, increasing lipid solubility increases anesthetic potency.

The water solubility (hydrophilic nature) of local anesthetics is primarily determined by the amine portion. An agent with a lower pKa will exist in

Table 1-1. Functional Characteristics of Local Anesthetics

	Lipid Solubility[a]	Potency[a]	Protein Binding[a]	Duration (min) Without Epinephrine	Duration (min) With Epinephrine
Procaine	0.6	1	5.8	15–30	30–90
Mepivacaine	1.0	2	77	30–120	60–400
Lidocaine	2.9	4	64	30–120	60–400
Chloroprocaine	N/A	4	N/A	30–60	N/A
Tetracaine	80	16	76	120–240	240–480
Bupivacaine	28	16	95	120–240	240–480
Etidocaine	141	16	94	200	240–360

[a] Relative values.
Abbreviation: N/A, not applicable.
(Data from Covino and Vassallo, 1976.)

body fluids with fewer charged molecules. Agents in the base form (un-charged) will diffuse across cell membranes more easily, thereby resulting in quicker onset of action. Once across the membrane, however, it is the positively charged (cationic) form that actively binds to membrane receptors.

The anesthetic receptors within the nerve cell membrane are thought to be proteins. Affinity of the anesthetic agent for these receptors is important in determining duration of action. Both ends of the anesthetic molecule partici-pate in protein binding activity.

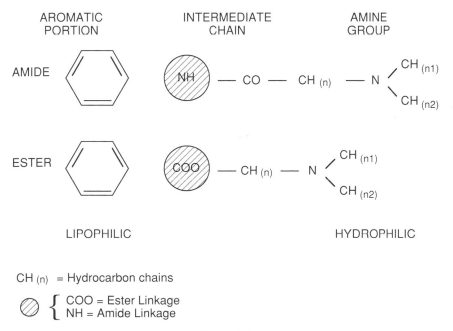

Figure 1-2

2

Anesthetic Agents

WHICH ANESTHETIC AGENT TO CHOOSE?

The choice of anesthetic should be tailored to the procedure being considered and to patient sensitivities. Biopsies and other quick procedures require an anesthetic with a short onset of action. The duration of the anesthetic agent is less important. If planning a larger procedure requiring nerve blocks, it is preferable to choose an agent with a longer duration of action, one at least as long as the time required for the procedure. Anesthetic agents are available in a variety of concentrations. Generally, the higher concentrations are reserved for nerve blocks. If it is planned to anesthetize a large area of skin a lower concentration of the anesthetic should be considered, in order to avoid exceeding the maximum allowable dose. Another point to consider is that the amide-type anesthetics have a much lower incidence of allergy compared with the ester-type anesthetics and are thus considered the first-line drugs of choice. For most dermatologic procedures, 1 percent lidocaine with epinephrine at $1:200,000$ offers the best combination of rapid onset of action, reasonably long duration, and safety. When one is doing a procedure requiring an agent with a longer duration of action, choices include bupivacaine and etidocaine. As a general rule, longer-acting anesthetics are more toxic and thus have a lower maximal safe dosage.

Presently, there are two major classes of local anesthetic agents, which are based on their chemical structure: esters and amides. Agents falling into a particular classification share characteristics related to allergy and metabolism (Table 2-1 and see Table 1-1).

When choosing an anesthetic, it is sometimes important to keep in mind the method by which the anesthetic agents are metabolized. This is important in avoiding potential toxicity. The metabolism of a particular agent depends on the structure of the intermediate chain that comprises the agent (see Fig. 1-2).

ESTER-TYPE LOCAL ANESTHETICS

Ester-type anesthetics contain an ester linkage, which is hydrolyzed by the plasma enzyme pseudocholinesterase (see Fig. 1-2). Patients with a rare genetic defect in the structure of this enzyme may be unable to metabolize

5

Table 2-1. Common Available Local Anesthetics

Generic	Proprietary	Concentrations (%)
Ester Class (plasma metabolism)		
Cocaine		2 to 10 (topical)
Procaine	Novocain	0.5, 1.0, 2.0
Chloroprocaine	Nesacaine	0.5, 1.0, 2.0
Tetracaine	Pontocaine	0.1, 0.25 (0.5 ophthalmic)
Amide Class (liver metabolism)		
Lidocaine	Xylocaine	0.5, 1.0, 2.0 (2.0, 5.0 topical)
Mepivacaine	Carbocaine	1.0, 2.0
Prilocaine	Citanest	1.0, 2.0, 3.0
Bupivacaine	Marcaine/Sensorcaine	0.25, 0.5, 0.75
Etidocaine	Duranest	0.5, 1.0

an ester-type local anesthetic, which raises the potential for toxicity from elevated blood levels. Ester-type anesthetics are metabolized to para-aminobenzoic acid (PABA), which inhibits the action of sulfonamides. Of the ester-type local anesthetic agents, procaine, tetracaine, and cocaine are the most frequently used.

Cocaine

Cocaine is an effective topical anesthetic, particularly for procedures involving the mucosal surfaces of the nose or mouth. It is a unique topical agent in that it also possesses vasoconstrictor activity, which is helpful in these areas. It is usually used as a 2 to 10 percent solution. The onset of action is from 3 to 5 minutes using a 4 percent solution. Since topical application can have systemic side effects, including hypertension, tachycardia, and central nervous system (CNS) excitation, cocaine should be used with caution in patients with hypertension, severe cardiovascular disease, or uncontrolled hyperthyroidism. Use in the eye is contraindicated since clouding of the cornea with ulceration may result. Because of the potential problems with its use, cocaine has been replaced by other agents for topical anesthesia. It is no longer available for internal use because of systemic side effects.

Procaine (Novocaine)

Procaine has a quick onset of action but a short duration. It penetrates tissue poorly and is not effective topically on mucous membranes. Hydrolyzed in the body to PABA, procaine should not be used in patients allergic to PABA or procaine penicillin. It is available in concentrations of 0.5 percent, 1 percent and 2 percent, with or without epinephrine at 1:200,000. Yellow discoloration of the solution can occur and is harmless. This agent has generally been replaced by lidocaine.

Tetracaine (Pontocaine)

Tetracaine is markedly more potent than procaine and therefore potentially more toxic. It has a slower onset of action, but it has the longest duration of any of the ester-type anesthetics. Like procaine, tetracaine is a PABA derivative. A 1 to 2 percent solution can be used as a topical anesthetic on mucosal surfaces. A 0.5 percent ophthalmic preparation is also available. Overzealous use of this agent on mucous membranes has been associated with systemic toxicity. Tetracaine is available for injection in concentrations of 0.1 and 0.25 percent, with or without epinephrine. Due to the higher risk of allergy, it has been generally replaced by bupivacaine or etidocaine as a long-acting anesthetic for dermatology.

Chloroprocaine (Nesacaine)

Chloroprocaine is rarely used in dermatology, as injection into the skin is accompanied by an uncomfortable burning sensation, which is due to the acidity of the solution. Its anesthetic potency is somewhat greater than that of procaine and it has the advantage of having the shortest duration of action of the local anesthetic agents. Because of this latter point, some physicians consider chloroprocaine the safest agent for use in very ill patients, although the burning sensation experienced with it can be quite anxiety-provoking. A 0.5, 1.0, or 2.0 percent solution, with or without epinephrine, can be used for infiltrative anesthesia. Exposure to light can turn solutions brown, rendering them ineffective. Chloroprocaine is not effective topically.

AMIDE-TYPE LOCAL ANESTHETICS

The amide local anesthetics have a very low incidence of allergy and are generally considered safer than the ester-type anesthetics. Amide local anesthetics are primarily metabolized by microsomal enzymes located in the liver. Caution must be exercised in patients with severe liver disease, as they may be at increased risk of toxic effects of agents of this class. β-Blockers may decrease blood flow to the liver, which can also lead to a diminution of the metabolism of amide local anesthetics. If an amide-type anesthetic must be used in treatment of a patient with severe liver disease, a smaller dose should be given.

Lidocaine, mepivacaine, bupivacaine, and etidocaine are the most frequently used amide anesthetics.

Lidocaine (Xylocaine)

Lidocaine has a more rapid onset and a longer, more intense anesthetic activity than procaine. It penetrates the tissue readily and has become the standard medium-duration anesthetic. Lidocaine is effective topically on mucous membranes and is available as a 2 or 5 percent gel or ointment. Lidocaine is reported to produce sleepiness on rare occasions. The injectable form is available in concentrations with or without epinephrine of 0.5 percent, 1.0 percent (used for local infiltration) and 2.0 percent (useful for nerve blocks).

Mepivacaine

Mepivacaine is slightly more rapid in onset and longer in duration of action than lidocaine. It is reported to produce less vasodilation experimentally than other anesthetic agents, thereby negating the need to use epinephrine. We have not found this to be the case in our practice; wound bleeding with mepivacaine appears similar to that of other agents without epinephrine. Since mepivacaine is less toxic than lidocaine and has a higher maximal safe dose, it may be advantageous to use it when larger amounts of anesthesia are required. It is not effective topically. For injection it is available in concentrations of 1 percent or 2 percent, with or without epinephrine. For general use, this agent offers little advantage over lidocaine.

Prilocaine (Citanest)

Prilocaine is a slowly absorbed agent with a slower onset of action, but a longer duration of action, than lidocaine. Its major drawback is dose-dependant methemoglobinemia and it should not be used in patients with pulmonary disease, congestive heart failure, or renal disease. There is little to recommend this agent over others available. It is prepared in concentrations of 1.0, 2.0 and 3.0 percent for injection.

Bupivacaine (Marcaine/Sensorcaine)

Bupivacaine is more potent than lidocaine, and has a longer duration of action. Its main disadvantage is a slow onset of action, which may be overcome by mixing it with an equal part of 2 percent lidocaine solution. Bupivacaine is particularly useful for nerve blocks, which can last over 4 hours with this agent. For local infiltration it offers little advantage over lidocaine with epinephrine. The addition of epinephrine to bupivacaine offers little increase in the duration of anesthesia. Bupivacaine is available in concentrations of 0.25, 0.5 and 0.75 percent, with or without epinephrine. It is not effective topically.

Etidocaine (Duranest)

Etidocaine is a long-acting anesthetic with advantages over bupivacaine, which include lower toxicity, a higher maximal safe dose, and a relatively short onset of action. The advantages make it an ideal agent when a long procedure is planned and epinephrine cannot be used (e.g., digital or penile block). It is available in concentrations of 0.5 percent and 1 percent, with or without epinephrine.

3

Toxicity of
Local Anesthetics

Local anesthetics are generally very safe drugs; it is rare for the dermatologist to encounter toxicity from local anesthetics during routine use. However, toxicity secondary to overdosage may be encountered by the dermatologic surgeon. The most common such setting is a procedure that involves a large area, and therefore requires larger quantities of anesthetic solution; such procedures include scalp reduction, skin flap reconstruction, hair transplantation, and liposuction. Improper use of anesthetics can also lead to toxicity. Thus, it is important that the dermatologist performing surgery be familiar with both the symptoms of anesthetic toxicity and the correct method of treating them should they occur. Proper technique and attention to the patient's medical history can greatly decrease the chances of a toxic reaction. Toxic side effects can be divided into local and systemic reactions.

LOCAL REACTIONS

Improper injection technique is the cause of many local reactions attributed to the anesthesic. Ecchymosis or hematoma formation caused by the laceration of blood vessels is a fairly frequent local reaction, particularly in vascular areas such as the head, neck, and genitalia. Ecchymosis is also more likely if the patient is taking aspirin or other anticoagulants or has a bleeding disorder.

Infection with abscess formation can occur at the site of injection. Infection is almost invariably due to neglect of proper sterile technique.

Nerve damage by needle laceration is uncommon during injection, but can occur, especially during peripheral nerve blocks. The elicitation of paresthesias during insertion of the needle indicates contact with a nerve and should be avoided in order to prevent nerve damage. Proper injection technique, which will be discussed later, can greatly reduce the risk of nerve damage.

Another potential cause of nerve damage is neurotoxicity from the anesthetic agent. Irreversible nerve damage has been reported with large doses of

9

chloroprocaine used for nerve blocks and with other agents used at high concentrations. The neurotoxicity is partly due to the low pH of the solution.

In general, most local anesthetics produce relatively little tissue reaction. However, tissue necrosis has been reported with epinephrine employed at concentrations exceeding 1 : 50,000. Such high concentrations of epinephrine are completely unnecessary; concentrations of 1 : 100,000 or less are equally effective in producing vasoconstriction and are much safer to use. Inadvertent injection of other toxic substances used in dermatology, such as sclerosing solution, can also produce tissue necrosis. Solution bottles should be clearly marked and routinely checked before use in order to prevent such accidental injections.

Pain is a local reaction considered to be an unfortunate but inevitable accompaniment of injectable local anesthesia. It is a composite of several factors, including acidity and other direct tissue toxicities relative to the agent, the needle stick, injection technique, and the patient's reaction. These factors can be controlled partially, thereby minimizing patient discomfort and anxiety. Methods of lessening the pain of injection are discussed later.

SYSTEMIC REACTIONS

Both low and high blood levels of local anesthetics may be associated with systemic reactions (Table 3-1).

Causes of High Blood Levels of Local Anesthetics

Overdosage During Procedures Involving a Large Area

Overdosage during procedures involving a large area is caused by exceeding the recommended dosage of a particular anesthetic agent (see Table 5-1). This can be avoided with the following steps:

1. Use the lowest dose necessary to induce anesthesia.
2. Before reinjecting an area, allow sufficient time for the anesthetic to work. This is particularly important when using agents with a slower onset of action.
3. Use epinephrine unless contraindicated.
4. Employ nerve blocks when possible.
5. When anesthetizing a large area, use the lowest effective concentration of anesthetic.

Intravenous Administration

Intravenous administration is probably the most common cause of elevated blood levels of local anesthetics; injection of as little as 10 mg of lidocaine (1 ml of 1 percent solution) into the cerebral circulation can induce toxic symptoms. This inadvertent event is particularly a problem when anesthetizing highly vascular areas (head, neck, or genitalia), injecting into inflamed

Table 3-1. Systemic Lidocaine Toxicity

		Signs	Treatment
Central nervous system	Early 1–5 μg/ml[a]	Tinnitus, circumoral pallor, metallic taste in mouth, lightheadedness, talkativeness, nausea, emesis, diplopia	Recognition, observation; no further lidocaine until resolved
	Mid 5–12 μg/ml[a]	Nystagmus, slurred speech, hallucinations, muscle twitching facial/hand tremors, seizures	Diazepam; airway maintenance; observation
	Late 20–25 μg/ml[a]	Apnea, coma	Respiratory support
Cardiovascular System	High blood levels	Myocardial depression, bradycardia, atrioventricular blockade, ventricular arrythmias, vasodilation, hypotension	Oxygen; vasopressors; cardiopulmonary resuscitation
Allergy		Pruritis, urticaria, angioedema, nausea, wheezing, anaphylaxis, ? anaphylactoid reactions	Antihistamines; epinephrine, 0.3 ml 1 : 1,000 SQ; oxygen; airway maintenance
Psychogenic		Pallor, diaphoresis, hyperventilation, lightheadedness, nausea, syncope	Trendelenberg position; cool compresses; observation
Pregnancy		Class B agent; immature fetal liver may not tolerate high doses	Avoid complex procedures, particularly in the first trimester

[a] Blood levels.

tissue, or performing nerve blocks in areas that contain large arteries. Intravenous administration can be avoided by careful technique and by aspiration before injection. It is traditionally stated that aspiration through a 30 gauge needle is unreliable and that a larger-diameter needle (25 gauge or larger) should be used. It is possible to obtain a blood return through small-gauge needles; however, a negative aspiration does not exclude the possibility that the needle tip is located in a vessel. A prudent approach in this situation would be to inject the anesthetic slowly while moving the needle slightly.

Impairment of Metabolism of the Anesthetic Agent

The metabolism of an agent depends on the structure of the intermediate chain of which it is composed.

Ester-type anesthetics are hydrolyzed by the plasma enzyme pseudocholinesterase. Persons with deficient pseudocholinesterase activity may be limited in their ability to hydrolyze an ester-type local anesthetic, which results in toxicity due to elevated blood levels.

The metabolism of the amid-type local anesthetics is primarily by microsomal enzymes located in the liver. Potentially toxic blood levels may therefore occur in patients with severe liver disease. Any condition that decreases blood flow to the liver, such as heart failure or administration of β-blockers, also decreases the metabolism of amide-type local anesthetics. In such a patient, if an amide-type anesthetic is used, the smallest dose possible should be given and the patient should be carefully monitored for signs of toxicity.

Effects of High Blood Levels of Local Anesthetics

High blood levels of local anesthetics acutely affect primarily the central nervous system (CNS) and the cardiovascular system.

Central Nervous System

The CNS is sensitive to elevated blood levels of local anesthetics. Inhibitory neurons of the cerebral cortex are the first to be suppressed. Their suppression results in unchecked activity of excitatory neurons, which produces stimulatory signs and symptoms in a dose-related fashion.

Symptoms of CNS toxicity occurring at low blood levels (1 to 5 μg/ml lidocaine) that have been noted during routine dermatologic procedures, such as hair transplantation, include the following:

Ringing in the ears
Circumoral numbness and tingling
Metallic taste in the mouth
Lightheadedness
Talkativeness
Nausea and vomiting
Double vision

At moderate blood levels (5 to 8 μg/ml lidocaine) the following prodromal signs of seizure activity can be seen:

Nystagmus
Slurred speech
Hallucinations
Localized muscle twitching
Fine tremors of the face and hands

At blood levels of 8 to 12 μg/ml lidocaine, seizure activity can be observed. Focal seizure activity is initially observed. This may increase to culminate into grand mal seizures, which can be fatal if they are not treated. Fortunately, most seizure activity due to local anesthetics is self-limiting, due to redistribution and metabolism of the drug. Possible exceptions to this rule are the longer-acting anesthetic agents (tetracaine, bupivacaine, and etidocaine). Preoperative sedation with 10 mg of diazepam has been shown to increase the threshold at which seizure activity occurs.

At extremely high blood levels (20 to 25 μg/ml of lidocaine), the excitatory neurons become depressed and respiratory depression followed by coma may result.

A blood level of 1 μg/ml can result from the intravenous administration of 50 mg of lidocaine (5 ml of 1 percent solution). CNS toxicity correlates with the potency of the anesthetic; more potent local anesthetics (bupivacaine and etidocaine) induce CNS toxicity at much lower blood levels. CNS toxicity is also more likely to occur in patients taking phenytoin (Dilantin).

TREATMENT OF SEIZURES INDUCED BY LOCAL ANESTHETICS

Seizures induced by local anesthetics should be treated with the following measures:

1. Lie the patient flat in a supine position and protect the patient against injury.
2. Maintain an airway and offer ventilatory support if necessary. Hyperventilation increases the cortical seizure threshold.
3. Delivery of oxygen. This is best accomplished with a mask.
4. Intravenous diazepam. This should be reserved for sustained seizure activity. Five to 10 mg should be administered slowly, (at a rate of 1 to 2 mg/min) until seizures cease. Since the duration of activity is short (15 to 20 minutes), other treatment should be started, especially if seizures are caused by long-acting anesthetics. (see Applegate and Fox, Suggested Readings).

Certain anesthetic agents, such as lidocaine and prilocaine, tend to induce sleepiness. This side effect has been observed at doses occasionally used in dermatologic surgery.

Cardiovascular System

Cardiovascular side effects during local anesthesia are primarily caused by the stimulatory effects of epinephrine. In general, the cardiovascular system is more resistant to the toxic effects of local anesthetics than the CNS. However, high blood levels of local anesthetics, particularly the more potent agents bupivacaine and etidocaine, can directly depress myocardial contractility, thereby leading to hypotension. This may be compounded by a direct vasodilatory effect of the anesthetic. Higher blood levels can lead to atrioventricular block, bradycardia, and ventricular arrhythmias. These effects probably occur more commonly in patients with conduction disturbances requiring antiarrhythmic medications. These cardiac side effects have generally been associated with the intravascular injection of high doses of anesthetics. Oxygen, vasopressors, and cardiopulmonary resuscitation should be administered as treatment.

Pregnancy

Local anesthetics can cross the placenta and are considered class B agents. Although there is little evidence of human fetal toxicity, as with any drug it is wise to avoid the use of local anesthetics, particularly during the first trimester, when organogenesis has begun. The hepatic system of the fetus is less able to handle the metabolism of amid-type anesthetic agents. Therefore, large-area procedures requiring local anesthesia should be postponed until after delivery. Since small procedures, such as biopsies and simple excisions, require minimal amounts of anesthesic, risks to the fetus are probably negligible. Treatment of possibly malignant lesions therefore should not be delayed.

Breast Feeding

All local anesthetics are excreted into breast milk to some extent and toxicity to the infant is possible if a large amount of anesthetic is used. Thus, it is best to avoid performing unnecessary elective procedures while a woman is breast feeding.

Effects of Low Blood Levels of Anesthesia

Allergy

Systemic reactions that may be associated with low blood levels include allergy and idiosyncratic responses.

Less than 1 percent of all reactions to local anesthetics are allergic in nature. True allergy to the amide class of anesthetics is exceedingly rare, although the ester-type local anesthetics carry a definite risk of allergic reaction. Many patients with allergy to local anesthetics have a history of allergy to other substances. Allergic reactions may be classified as either type I (immediate or anaphylactic) or type IV (delayed hypersensitivity).

TYPE I REACTIONS

Type I reactions occur most frequently with the ester group of local anesthetics. The metabolic product, para-aminobenzoic acid (PABA), is highly allergenic. Cross-reactivity occurs among the various ester-type anesthetics and with methylparabens, a preservative found in multiple-dose vials. Patients allergic to procaine penicillin may also cross-react with procaine.

The amide group of local anesthetics do not cross-react with the ester class. Allergy to amide-type agents is rare. When an allergic reaction occurs with the use of amide-type anesthetics, it is usually due to the preservatives, methylparabens, and sodium metabisulfite found in multiple-dose vials. If this occurs, unpreserved single-dose vials of lidocaine are available. Lidocaine used in the treatment of cardiac arrhythmias (2 percent concentration) has no preservatives.

Anesthetics containing metabisulfite should be avoided in patients reporting sensitivity to sulfites.

Prodromal symptoms of anaphylaxis include the following:

Skin: pruritus, urticaria, erythema, facial swelling
Gastrointestinal: nausea, vomiting, abdominal cramps, diarrhea
Respiratory: coughing, wheezing, dyspnea, cyanosis, laryngeal edema

Treatment of Type I Reactions
Type I reactions should be treated in the following manner:

1. Epinephrine is the drug of choice for initial treatment.
   For less severe reactions, use 0.3 to 0.5 mg (0.3 to 0.5 ml of 1 : 1,000 solution) SQ q 20 to 30 minutes, up to three doses. Injection into the site the anesthetic was administered may delay absorption of the antigen.
   For treatment of anaphylaxis, use 0.5 mg (5 ml of 1 : 10,000 solution) IV repeated q 5 to 10 minutes as needed. If an intravenous line is not available, sublingual or endotracheal administration using 1 : 1000 solution should be tried.
2. Maintain a patent airway.
3. Deliver oxygen.
4. Transport the patient to an acute care facility. All patients experiencing an acute type I reaction should be observed for at least 6 hours.

TYPE IV REACTIONS

Delayed hypersensitivity from topical use has been reported to both ester and amide classes of anesthetics and is much more common than type I allergy. There is no relationship between type IV hypersensitivity to the amide-type of local anesthetics and type I reaction as determined by intradermal tests performed on patients with type IV sensitivity to these agents. Anaphylaxis can occur with topical administration. Contact dermatitis to topical anesthetics is treated with either topical or systemic steroids, depending on the severity of the reaction.

PSYCHOGENIC REACTIONS

Most patients who report a history of allergic reaction to local anesthesics probably experienced a vasovagal reaction, which may be psychogenic in nature. This response may result from a patient's fear of needles or may occur as a reaction to the pain of injection. Symptoms include pallor, diaphoresis, hyperventilation, lightheadedness, nausea, and syncope.

Treatment of Vasovagal Reaction

1. Lower the head and elevate the legs to correct the effects of postural hypotension. Do not leave the patient unattended.
2. Turn the head to the side should vomiting occur.
3. Smelling salts (ammonia capsules) may be used to arouse the patient.

Mentally preparing the patient for the injection and careful injection technique can go a long way in reducing the possibility of a vasovagal response. Since this is always a possibility with any patient it is essential that the patient lie down during the injection.

AN APPROACH TO THE PATIENT REPORTING ALLERGY TO LOCAL ANESTHETICS

It is difficult by history alone to differentiate between true allergic reaction and psychogenic reactions. Controversy exists as to the diagnostic value of skin testing in determining if a particular drug is responsible for an acute anaphylactic reaction. Both false-positive and false-negative reactions are possible, and a negative test result does not exclude the possibility of a similar reaction occurring again. If the reaction is allergic in nature, skin testing is probably more useful in detecting the specific agent responsible for the reaction than other methods, such as basophil degranulation tests or radioimmunoassay.

Several methods of challenge testing using serial titration exist (see Suggested Readings). These methods differ as to whether or not suspected agents are diluted before injection. Testing should be performed within 3 months of the event, since reliability of the method decreases after this time. Patients should have ceased taking any drugs that may interfere with the response, such as antihistamines, sympathomimetics, steroids, theophyllines, and disodium cromoglycate.

Ampules containing cardiac-grade, preservative-free lidocaine are available for testing. If the dilution method is used, saline free of preservatives should be the diluent. Since reactions to preservatives present in multiple-dose vials of local anesthetics such as parabens and metabisulfite are possible, these should be tested separately.

Skin testing is performed with a 1 ml syringe capped with a 26 gauge needle. The generation of a wheal greater than 1.0 cm in diameter arising within 10 minutes of the injection and lasting at least 30 minutes with a negative reaction at the control site is generally regarded as a positive response. Skin testing is easy to perform but evaluation does require experience and should always be done with cardiovascular support readily available. If this is not available, consideration should be given to the use of alternative agents.

Alternative Agents for Patients Reporting Allergy to Local Anesthetics

Normal Saline (0.9 percent)

Intradermal injection of 0.9 percent saline can produce temporary anesthesia, during which time procedures such as small punch or shave biopsies may be performed. The anesthetic effect is due to physical pressure on the nerve endings, and persists as long as the skin remains distended and blanched. There may be a contribution to this effect by the presence of benzyl alcohol as a preservative in some saline preparations. If it is possible that the patient is sensitive to the preservative methylparabens, nonbacteriostatic saline should be used.

Antihistamines

Diphenhydramine (Benadryl) and other injectable antihistamines have been employed as injectable local anesthetics. Although effective, these agents have the disadvantage of short half-life, sedation, painful injection, and reports of tissue necrosis. For these reasons they are usually used in a diluted form (diphenhydramine in dosages of 10 to 25 mg/ml). Most efficacious in short, simple procedures, they have been used successfully for procedures ranging from biopsies to Mohs surgery. Combination with epinephrine at 1:200,000 has been reported to enhance anesthetic potency. Because of the sedative side effect, patients should be cautioned not to drive for several hours afterward.

4

Vasoconstriction and the Use of Epinephrine

Local anesthetics, except cocaine, generally produce vascular smooth muscle relaxation, which results in vasodilation. This decreases the amount of active drug at the site of injection because of enhanced absorption. Thus, adding a vasoconstrictor to local anesthetic solutions has the following advantages:

1. *The absorption of the anesthetic is decreased.* This increases anesthetic efficiency, permitting use of smaller amounts of anesthetics.
2. *The duration of the anesthesia is prolonged.* The effect is greater in short-acting agents, such as lidocaine or procaine. Anesthetic duration of these agents may be doubled.
3. *There is a reduced risk of systemic toxicity.* The absorption rate is decreased, which allows the body additional time to metabolize the drug.
4. *Bleeding at the operative site is reduced.* This is particularly important when operating in highly vascular areas such as the head or neck.

The most widely used vasoconstrictor for local anesthesia is epinephrine. It is the most potent vasoconstrictor available. Other vasoconstrictors used occasionally include phenylephrine (Neo-Synephrine), levonordefrin (Neo-Cobefrin) and norepinephrine (Levofed).

EPINEPHRINE

Most local anesthetics are available premixed with epinephrine, usually at a concentration of 1 : 100,000 (1 mg/100 ml). Although this concentration of epinephrine is safe in most instances, it is advantageous at times to use the lowest concentration possible. We have found epinephrine at 1 : 200,000 equally effective in producing vasoconstriction adequate for most dermatologic procedures. Concentrations as low as 1:500,000 epinephrine have shown efficacy. Stronger solutions of epinephrine, 1:50,000 or greater offer no further advantage and increase the risk of tissue necrosis because of prolonged ischemia.

Epinephrine is less effective in prolonging the anesthetic properties of the longer-acting anesthetics such as bupivacaine and etidocaine, which are already highly tissue-bound.

Epinephrine is degraded by ultraviolet light, heat, oxygen, and alkaline pH. For this reason, epinephrine-containing solutions are prepared at an acidic pH with antioxidants, in order to increase the shelf life of the epinephrine. Solutions should be discarded if they are discolored or contain a precipitate.

The intradermal injection of lidocaine produces almost immediate anesthesia. However, it usually takes 7 to 15 minutes for the full vasoconstrictive effect of epinephrine to be achieved. For this reason, it is advisable to wait approximately 15 minutes after injecting epinephrine, especially in highly vascular areas or when large-area procedures are contemplated. Vasoconstriction is recognized clinically as blanching of the overlaying skin.

A potential problem is delayed bleeding after the epinephrine effect wears off. This could lead to the possible formation of a hematoma. Good intraoperative hemostasis and appropriate pressure dressings minimize this problem.

ALTERNATE VASOCONSTRICTORS

Phenylephrine is a less potent vasoconstrictor than epinephrine, therefore requiring use at higher concentrations (1:20,000 to 1:50,000). It has a longer duration of action than epinephrine. Cardiac side effects such as tachycardia occur less frequently, as phenylephrine has minimal effect on the myocardium. Its major advantage over epinephrine is that it can induce vasoconstriction topically on mucous membranes. It is available for topical use as a 0.5 percent solution or gel. Concentrations greater than this can result in significant pressor effects.

Levonordefrin (Neo-Cobefrin) and *norepinephrine* (Levofed) are occasionally used in local anesthesia. Levonordefrin is a more stable, but less potent alternative to epinephrine and is usually used at a concentration of 1:20,000. Norepinephrine is occasionally available premixed with an anesthetic at a concentration of 1:80,000.

ADVERSE EFFECTS FROM VASOCONSTRICTORS

Local Effects

Pain

Pain upon injection is the most common local side effect when epinephrine is used. It is predominantly related to the acidity of epinephrine-containing solutions. Commercially prepared lidocaine with epinephrine is available at a pH of 3.5 to 4.5. Plain lidocaine, without epinephrine, can be prepared at a higher pH (6.5 to 6.8). Injection of acidic solutions can result in temporary tissue acidosis and pain. It is this difference in pH that is responsible for the increased pain experienced by patients who receive lidocaine with epinephrine as compared with those who receive plain lidocaine. There are several methods of reducing this pain (see Ch. 10).

Tissue Necrosis

Tissue necrosis from the use of epinephrine is a possibility, although it is infrequently seen in general practice. The use of epinephrine in areas supplied with end arteries, such as the digits and penis, has tradionally been avoided due to reports of tissue necrosis. Patients at particular risk for this usually have an underlying vascular disease, which may be due to smoking, diabetes mellitus, peripheral vascular disease, scleroderma, or other vasospastic disease. Since in practice it is difficult to predict which patients have a compromised vasculature, it is prudent to avoid the use of epinephrine in these areas.

Wound Healing

Wound healing reportedly is adversely affected by epinephrine. We have not found this is be clinically significant for most dermatologic procedures. Reports of flap necrosis secondary to the use of epinephrine are more likely due to improper flap design or chronic tobacco abuse by the patient.

Delayed Postoperative Bleeding

Delayed postoperative bleeding is another adverse local effect, as discussed in the earlier section on epinephrine.

Systemic Effects

Systemic adverse reactions from the use of epinephrine predominantly affect the cardiovascular and central nervous systems (CNS); such an effect is most commonly seen as mild transient tachycardia associated with an excited state in the patient. This can occur with as little as 2 ml of an anesthetic containing epinephrine at 1 : 100,000 concentration. If a larger amount of anesthetic solution containing epinephrine is injected, this reaction can progress to palpitations, sweating, pallor, chest pain, tremors, nervousness, headaches, and hypertension, which are usually seen within 4 minutes of injection. Hypertension does not usually occur in normal individuals until at least 0.5 mg (50 ml of 1 : 100,000 solution) of epinephrine is injected. The occurrence of severe systemic side effects is most commonly due to intravascular injection of the anesthetic.

The maximum dose of epinephrine injected in normal individuals should not exceed 1 mg at any one time. This is the equivalent to 100 ml of 1 : 100,000 solution. As much as 10 percent of patients receiving injection of a local

Table 4-1. Systemic Epinephrine Toxicity

	Signs	Treatment
Central nervous system	Nervousness, headaches, tremors May precipate psychiatric episode in predisposed patients	Restrict further dose; diazepam
Cardiovascular system	Tachycardia, palpitations, chest pain, hypertension; ECG abnormalities	Vasodilators: hydralazine, clonidine, sublingual nifedipine
Pregnancy	Reduced placental blood flow May induce labor in the third trimester	Avoid use if possible

anesthetic with epinephrine show electrocardiographic (ECG) changes; however, most are of little consequence. Patients with a history of heart disease are at higher risk for the development of significant arrhythmias or angina with epinephrine. At particular risk for this are patients with unstable angina or those who have cardiac arrhythmias requiring medication. If epinephrine must be used in such patients, it should be at a concentration of 1 : 300,000. The New York Heart Association suggests a maximal dose of 0.2 mg (20 ml of 1 : 100,000 epinephrine) in patients with cardiac disease (Table 4-1).

CONTRAINDICATIONS TO THE USE OF EPINEPHRINE

The use of epinephrine is contraindicated in patients with pheochromocytoma, hyperthyroidism, severe hypertension, or cardiac disease. The relative contraindications to the use of epinephrine are numerous (Table 4-2). Epinephrine may be used safely in patients with cardiac disease, if absolutely necessary, as long as the total dose is kept low. When employing epinephrine in patients for whom there is a relative contraindication, we use a concentration of 1 : 300,000 or 1 : 400,000.

Table 4-2. Contraindications to Epinephrine

Contraindication	Comment
Severe hypertension	Dilute epinephrine in controlled hypertension, monitor frequently
Severe cardiovascular disease	Stimulates heart; peripheral vasodilation
Severe peripheral vascular occlusive disease	May cause distal ischemia—dilute epinephrine or do not use.
Hyperthyroidism, pheochromocytoma	May cause hypertension in uncontrolled disease
Relative Contraindications	**Comment**
Psychologic instability	May precipitate acute psychotic episode in predisposed patients
Pregnancy	First trimester: may interfere with organogenesis Third trimester: may induce labor
Propanolol (β-blockers)	Unopposed alpha stimulation—seen with as little as 8 ml lidocaine with epinephrine
Distal extremities, penis	Prolonged ischemia, necrosis

Pregnancy

The use of epinephrine during pregnancy, especially during the first or last trimester, is generally considered contraindicated by most obstetricians. During the first trimester, fetoplacental ischemia can theoretically effect organogenesis. In late pregnancy, placental ischemia by the systemic absorption of epinephrine may induce premature labor. For these reasons, it is wise to avoid the use of epinephrine during pregnancy. If epinephrine is considered necessary in a procedure, it should be used in dilute concentrations (e.g., 1 : 300,000).

EPINEPHRINE/β-BLOCKER INTERACTION

In patients taking β-blockers, injections of epinephrine may result in a potentially dangerous reaction. Epinephrine has α-1, β-1, and β-2 activity. α-1 Activity produces vasoconstriction; β-2 stimulation produces vasodilatation. β-1 Stimulation of the heart is both inotropic and chronotropic. Epinephrine administered systemically tends to lower blood pressure, since the β-2 vasodilatory effects tend to predominate. The injection of epinephrine in a patients taking β-blocker results in unopposed α-1 vasoconstriction. This can lead to paradoxic hypertension, which is followed by reflex bradycardia. The bradycardia may ultimately lead to cardiac arrest, and the extreme hypertension may lead to stroke. This reaction has occurred with as little as 8 ml of lidocaine with 1 : 200,000 dilution of epinephrine, in a patient taking 60 mg of propranalol daily. Treatment of this medical emergency is with intravenous chlorpromazine (given in 1 mg increments up to 5 mg) or a hydralazine drip (20 mg in 250 ml normal saline). Close monitoring is necessary.

Most dermatologic procedures employ small amounts of anesthetic, and therefore epinephrine/β-blocker interaction is not usually clinically apparent. However, for procedures requiring larger amounts of anesthesia, it is advisable to discuss the possibility of stopping β-blocker therapy with the patient's primary physician. This must be done gradually, since the abrupt discontinuation of β-blockers can induce angina. If this is not possible, we routinely

Table 4-3. β-Blockers Available in the U.S. (1990)

Generic	Proprietary	Manufacturer
Atenolol	Tenormin	ICI Pharmaceuticals
Penbutolol sulfate	Levatol	Reed & Carnrick
Metroprolol tartrate	Lopressor	Geigy
Carteolol HCl	Cartrol	Abbott
Esmolol HCl	Brevibloc	Dupont Critical Care
Betaxolol HCl	Kerlone	Searle
Acebutolol HCl	Sectral	Wyeth-Ayerst
Nadolol	Corgard	Princeton Pharmaceuticals
Pindolol	Visken	Sandoz
Timolol maleate	Blocadren	Merck, Sharp & Dohme
Propranolol HCl	Inderal	Ayerst
	Ipran	Major

dilute the anesthetic solution with plain lidocaine to achieve a 1 : 300,000 concentration of epinephrine. This has been used successfully on patients receiving a moderate to high degree of β-blockade. It is very important to monitor frequently blood pressure of patients taking propanolol or other β-blockers (Table 4-3).

5

Dosage of Lidocaine

Table 5-1 shows formulae for determining the maximum amount of lido-caine that can be safely injected at one time. Greater amounts of anesthetic can be injected when epinephrine is used, since it slows the rate of systemic absorption and therefore allows the body more time to metabolize the anesthetic. However, as with any drug, the least amount necessary to achieve the desired effect is recommended. There is evidence to suggest that preoperative use of diazepam can increase a patient's tolerance against anesthesia-induced seizures. This, however, does not affect the likelihood of occurrence of other dose-related phenomena.

Table 5-1 Lidocaine Dosing Recommendations[a,b] (1 percent Solution = 10 mg/ml)

	With Epinephrine	Without Epinephrine
Adults (150 lbs, 70 kg)	7.0 mg/kg; 500 mg total (50 ml)	4.5 mg/kg; 300 mg total (30 ml)
Children	3–4 mg/kg	1.5–2.5 mg/kg
	Suggest 0.5% lidocaine when large amounts required	

[a] See package inserts or *Physician's Desk Reference* for dosing information of other agents.
[b] Recommendations assume normal liver function and one-time injection. Additional lidocaine may be added during long procedures as metabolism proceeds.

6

Equipment

Proper equipment is important in providing efficient delivery of local anesthesia.

GLOVES

Gloves should always be worn when inducing local anesthesia. An injection is an invasive procedure carrying the risk of exposure to blood-borne diseases such as hepatitis and acquired immunodeficiency syndrome (AIDS). Boxes of clean, not necessarily sterile gloves should be readily available in operating areas. Latex gloves are preferred to vinyl gloves, as they permit better tactile sensation.

ALCOHOL

The skin should always be cleansed with either 70 percent ethyl or isopropyl alcohol before injection. There are reports of infection with abscess formation after anesthetic injection. This can be avoided completely if a few seconds are taken to cleanse the skin. Alcohol pledgets are convenient.

SYRINGES

Luer-lok syringes should be used (Figure 6-1). They provide a threaded sheath around the tip of the syringe that allows the needle hub to be screwed into place. This is particularly important when injecting into areas where there is dense tissue with little room for expansion, such as the nose, scalp, palms, and soles. Injection into these areas can cause back pressure on the anesthetic solution, which may cause the needle to separate from the syringe if the needle is not locked into place. Disposable plastic syringes are inexpensive and more than adequate for most procedures. Several sizes of syringes should be available. The size of syringe to use depends on the procedure being performed and the area being injected. Smaller syringes are easier to inject with, especially into dense tissues. However, in procedures requiring large amounts of anesthetic, a larger syringe will require less refills and be more efficient.

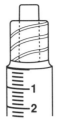

Luer-Lok Syringe

Figure 6-1

The following sizes of syringes should be on hand:

1 to 3 cc syringes. These are useful for biopsies or small excisions.
5 to 10 cc syringes. These are useful for nerve blocks or moderate-to-large-sized excisions. The 5 cc syringe may be easier to use especially in areas where there is little room for expansion, such as the scalp or soles, even if the procedure is large.
20 cc syringes. These are used for anesthetizing large areas such as the back or extremities.
Refilling syringes (McGhan). These, such as the McGhan syringe, are especially useful when anesthetizing large areas, such as when performing

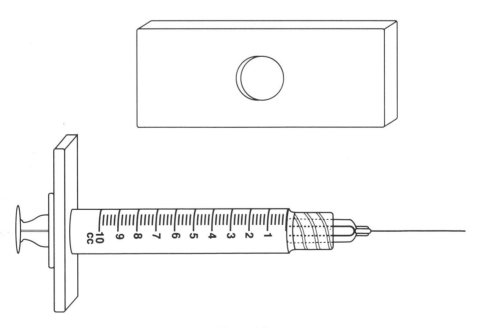

Figure 6-2

liposuction using the wet technique. With the McGhan syringe, large areas can be anesthetized quickly and easily. This syringe is usually connected to an intravenous bag containing a dilute anesthetic solution (see Ch. 11).

FINGER LEVERAGE PLATES

Finger leverage plates slip over the barrel of the syringe to increase the surface area of the flanges of the syringe. More power can be delivered to the plunger, which is helpful when injecting into areas with little room for expansion such as the scalp. They are usually made of Plexiglas and are available from a number of different manufacturers (Figure 6-2). Three ring disposable syringes are also available from Becton-Dickinson (Figure 6-3).

CARTRIDGES

Cartridges provide an alternate system for delivering local anesthesia (Figure 6-4). A variety of local anesthetics (e.g., Carbocaine) are available in disposable cartridges that screw into a metal syringe. These reusable syringes are often of the three-ring finger configuration or with wide-finger flanges. The

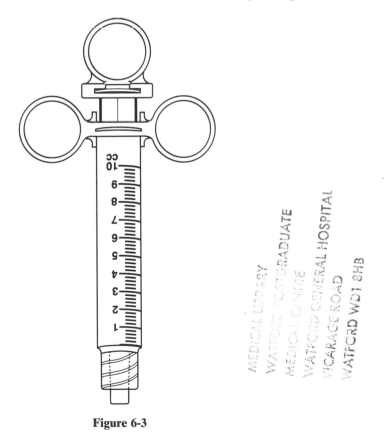

Figure 6-3

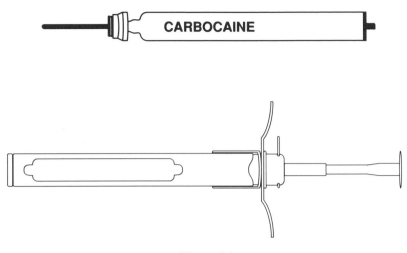

Figure 6-4

cartridges themselves are narrow-barreled and contain a small anesthetic volume (1.8 cc). While this system is easy to inject with, the small volume and increased expense may make the use of cartridges less attractive and less convenient.

NEEDLES

A variety of needles should be available. The types most useful for dermatology are discussed below.

30 Gauge

Anesthesia for most dermatologic surgical procedures is best delivered with a 30 gauge needle. Both $\frac{1}{2}$ and 1 inch lengths are available. The longer needle is particularly useful when a larger area needs to be anesthetized, since it can be threaded underneath the skin, thereby limiting the number of puncture sites. It is difficult to thread the longer needle into regions where the tissue is firm (scalp, palms, soles). When using finer-gauge needles it is wise to withdraw them to a more superficial plane before changing direction, since breakage can occur. Caution should be used when employing a 30 gauge needle for nerve blocks in which intravascular injection is a possibility. Aspiration of blood through a 30 gauge needle is less reliable than with larger-diameter needles.

25 Gauge

The 25 gauge needle is useful in areas of thick, firm skin such as the scalp, palms, and soles. Some advise its use when performing nerve blocks in vascular areas, where it is important to aspirate prior to injecting.

Spinal Needles

Spinal needles are long needles (3 inches and longer) that are particularly useful when injecting large areas. They limit the number of surface needle pokes and speed the injection procedure. They may be employed when performing a ring block on the scalp or trunk or before harvesting large split thickness skin grafts. They can be quite helpful when anesthetizing a large area for lipotransfer or liposuction using the refilling syringe. The needle sizes most applicable to these procedures are 22 and 25 gauge.

18 to 20 Gauge

Anesthesia can be most easily drawn into syringes from multiple-dose vials with larger gauge needles.

Disposal of Needles

Recapping of needles is potentially dangerous and is the most common cause of needlestick injury. If possible, needles should be discarded immediately after use by the physician in appropriate puncture-proof containers. Occasionally recapping is desirable. Recommendations for safely recapping needles are presented below.

DERMAJETS

The Dermajet permits injections without needles and may be useful in certain patients who have an extreme fear of needles. However, the Dermajet is painful and may be as anxiety-provoking for the patient as the proper use of a needle and syringe. Since the histology of tissue may be altered with the Dermajet, use of this device should be avoided when performing biopsies.

HYALURONIDASE

Hyaluronidase (Wydase) is a bovine-derived enzyme that modifies the permeability of connective tissue by hydrolyzing hyaluronic acid. When added to local anesthetic solutions it is reported to facilitate diffusion of anesthesia. It can double the anesthetic spread of lidocaine. This benefit is countered by a 50 percent shortening in the duration of anesthesia and a higher incidence of toxic reactions to anesthetic agents due to increased absorption. Since hyaluronidase is a foreign protein, allergic reactions to it are possible. The use of hyaluronidase is contraindicated in patients with an allergy to bee stings. For these reasons, hyaluronic acid has a limited role in a general dermatologic practice. Its use should be limited to situations in which it clearly offers a demonstrated advantage.

Hyaluronic acid is available in vials that, when reconstituted with saline, contain 150 United States Pharmacopeia (USP) U/ml. A useful dosage is 150 U/30 ml of anesthetic solution.

7

Topical Anesthetic Agents

Topical anesthesia can be useful in simple procedures and can be helpful in more complex procedures. To date, topical anesthesia can provide only superficial anesthesia down to the papillary dermis. Effectiveness on mucosal surfaces is much greater than on intact skin; absorption through mucous membranes is equivalent to intravenous dosing. Thus, a lower maximum dosage is recommended for topical use on mucous membranes. Patients should expectorate excess anesthetic to avoid excessive absorption. Even when anesthetizing only the labial or gingival mucosa it is possible to paralyze the gag reflex, secondary to swallowing small amounts of anesthetic. This reflex returns in approximately 15 minutes. The patient should be observed until function returns. The patient is advised not to eat or drink during this period, in order to avoid aspiration. The agents discussed below, have been useful in dermatology (Table 7-1).

COCAINE

Cocaine provides very reliable topical anesthesia on mucous membranes and is preferred by many otolaryngologists. Generally used as a 4 percent solution, it has the added advantage of producing vasoconstriction. The duration of anesthesia is 30 minutes and the maximum dosage at one sitting is 200 mg. However, because of the potential for abuse, it has been replaced in large part by other, safer agents.

BENZOCAINE

Use of benzocaine is generally limited to providing topical anesthesia on mucosal surfaces. It is available in a variety of forms, in concentrations ranging from 5 to 20 percent and can provide anesthesia for several hours. Of particular note is Cetacaine, which is an aerosol containing 14 percent benzocaine, 2 percent butyl aminobenzoate, and 2 percent tetracaine; it is widely used in otolaryngology. A 1 second spray releases 0.1 ml of solution and

Table 7-1. Topical Anesthetic Agents

Mucosal	
Cocaine	2–10% Solution
Benzocaine	5–20% Solution
Cetacaine	14% Benzocaine
	2% Butylaminobenzoate
	2% Tetracaine
Pontocaine	0.5% Tetracaine
Xylocaine	2, 5% Lidocaine jelly/ointment
Cutaneous	
Lidocaine	30%—Acid mantle cream
EMLA	Eutectic Mixture of Local Anesthesia
	2.5% Prilocaine
	2.5% Lidocaine
Refrigerant sprays	
Ethyl chloride	
Frigiderm	Dichlorotetrafluorethane
Fluroethyl	
Opthalmic	
Ophthane	0.5% Proparacaine
Ophthetic	
Pontocaine	0.5% Tetracaine
Dorsacaine	0.4% Benoxinate

produces anesthesia of mucosal surfaces in 30 seconds. Cetacaine does produce a temporary burning sensation when sprayed on the mucosa. Since the use of benzocaine is associated with a higher risk of contact allergy, in dermatology it has been generally replaced by lidocaine.

TETRACAINE

The potential toxicity from tetracaine limits its use in dermatology. A 0.5 percent topical solution is available for use on mucous membranes. It will provide anesthesia of the mucous membranes for up to 45 minutes. The maximum dosage is 50 mg. Patients who demonstrate contact allergy to benzocaine may cross-react with this product.

LIDOCAINE

Lidocaine is probably the safest topical anesthetic available to date. Available as a 2 percent or 5 percent jelly or ointment and as a 10 percent aerosol, it can provide reliable topical anesthesia on mucosal surfaces within 15 to 30 minutes. The maximum dosage on mucous membranes is 250 mg, and the duration of action is approximately 15 minutes. If vasoconstriction of mucosal surfaces is desired, lidocaine can be combined with phenylephrine (Neo-Synephrine), which is available as a 0.5 percent solution or jelly. This, however, does not increase the duration of action on mucosal surfaces. Anesthesia on intact skin surfaces is erratic and requires application times up to 2 hours under occlusion. Used in this manner, 30 percent lidocaine in acid mantle cream can provide anesthesia adequate to perform simple procedures.

EUTECTIC MIXTURE OF LOCAL ANESTHESIA

Eutectic mixture of local anesthesia (EMLA) is a topical anesthetic produced by Astra (Frolunda, Sweden), by combining 2.5 percent lidocaine cream with 2.5 percent prilocaine cream in their base forms. Application under occlusion for approximately 1 hour can provide superficial anesthesia to pinprick, allowing removal of superficial lesions. As of 1990 this has not been approved by the Food and Drug Administration (FDA), although it is available by direct order from Sweden.

REFRIGERANT SPRAYS

Refrigerant sprays have the advantage of inducing topical anesthesia within seconds on skin surfaces. Dichlorotetrafluoroethane (Frigiderm) and ethyl chloride can be used to freeze lesions such as seborrheic keratoses temporarily, permitting pain-free shave excision or curettage while the lesion remains frozen. The refrigerant is sprayed for 2 to 5 seconds, depending on the distance the can is held from the skin, until a white frost appears on the lesion. Prolonged freezing times should be avoided since hypopigmentation and atrophic scarring may result. Ethyl chloride is inflammable and explosive and should not be used with electrosurgical devices. Since ethyl chloride possesses general anesthetic properties, it should be sprayed in a direction away from the face. Liquid nitrogen can also be used as a topical anesthetic, but pain is usually produced because of its much lower temperature and it has a greater potential for postoperative discomfort and reaction.

Many dermatologists find refrigerant sprays helpful in immediately anesthetizing the skin surface just before inserting a needle. In this case, the skin surface only needs to be sprayed for 1 to 2 seconds, during which time the needle is inserted.

OPHTHALMIC ANESTHETICS

Local anesthetics prepared for injection often produce a burning sensation when placed on the conjunctival surface. For this reason ophthalmic preparations are recommended for topical anesthesia.

Proparacaine (Ophthane), 0.5 percent ophthalmic solution, is a very commonly used topical anesthetic for the eyes. One to two drops placed on the conjunctival surface will produce rapid anesthesia without irritation (Fig. 7-1). The duration of action is approximately 30 minutes. Application of this solution can help minimize patient discomfort during periocular procedures. With the conjunctival surface of the eyelid anesthetized, a needle can be painlessly introduced to anesthetize the remainder of the eyelid.

Other topical eye preparations include 0.5 percent tetracaine (Pontocaine) and 0.4 percent benoxinate (Dorsacaine). These agents cross-react with benzoic acid ester-type local anesthetics and should not be used in patients allergic to benzocaine. Proparacaine 0.5 percent (Ophthetic, Ophthane) is

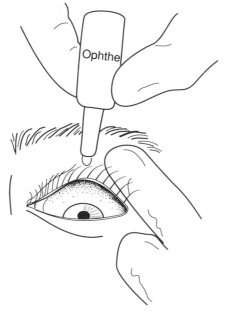

Figure 7-1

also a benzoic acid ester. However, due to differences in chemical structure it does not cross-react with the other agents. It also causes less eye irritation.

IONTOPHORESIS

The use of iontophoresis has been reported by Bezzant et al. to enhance the penetration of local anesthetic solutions (see Suggested Readings). With a 4 percent lidocaine solution with epinephrine at 1 : 50,000, the use of iontophoresis can induce topical anesthesia and vasoconstriction of skin surfaces within 7 minutes in a majority of patients. The effect can last up to 50 minutes. Although it may be useful in certain instances, the necessary use of an adhesive disk limits it application to rather small areas on flat surfaces.

8

Preoperative Sedatives and Other Adjuvant Agents

In certain patients it is desirable to use adjuvant therapy to induce local anesthesia. Children, particularly apprehensive patients, or patients undergoing more complex procedures may do well by receiving preoperative sedation. Although these agents are not capable of eliminating pain, they are helpful in calming the patient sufficiently to allow for the smooth induction of local anesthesia. As a general rule, all patients receiving sedation must be accompanied by a friend or family member who will drive the patient home.

It is imperative to inquire about other medications the patient is taking and prior experiences with sedative agents. Tolerance to preoperative sedatives varies greatly among patients. The elderly and patients with liver, thyroid, central nervous system, or pulmonary disease, and those with anemia can be quite sensitive to low doses of sedatives. Conversely, patients who smoke, regularly take sedatives or consume alcohol, or are extremely apprehensive often require higher dosing to achieve a similar effect. Children and the elderly can sometimes exhibit paradoxic agitation and delirium with sedatives. For these reasons, if sedatives are to be used, a pertinent medical history should be taken and resuscitative equipment should be available. Drug dosing depends on the patient's age, sex, weight, general physical and mental condition, and the type of procedure to be performed. The following is an abbreviated list of sedatives we have found safe and dependable.

BENZODIAZEPINES

Diazepam (Valium) and alprazolam (Xanax) are very effective antianxiety agents and are particularly useful in the patient who has an extraordinary fear of needles. Diazepam has a shorter onset of action and is generally preferred as a preoperative sedative. It has the additional advantage of inducing amnesia for the surgical procedure. Diazepam has also been shown to decrease the likelihood of anesthesia-induced seizures secondary to direct vascular injection or overdose. Sublingual administration allows a much more rapid onset of action than oral administration. Administration by either the oral or sublingual route is superior to intramuscular injection. The usual dosage of diazepam is 5 to 10 mg sublingually 30 minutes before operating, for adults, depending on the size and age of the patient. Intravenous administration is more effective and has a faster onset of action, but does require closer monitoring for respiratory depression.

Midazolam (Versed) is a useful agent, if parenteral administration is desired, due to its rapid onset of action. A dose of 5 mg IM (0.08 mg/kg) will induce sedation within 15 to 20 minutes. Although intravenous midazolam is more effective, it must be administered slowly as rapid injection can induce apnea, particularly in elderly patients. The usual initial intravenous dose is 2 mg, which is slowly titrated to the desired effect up to 0.15 mg/kg. Sedatives should be administered intravenously *only* by physicians familiar with the use of these drugs. The physician and office staff must be prepared to recognize and treat respiratory arrest should it occur.

Alprazolam is available only for oral administration. The usual dosage is 0.25 to 1.0 mg. These oral agents are also effective as hypnotics that can be prescribed for the evening before, allowing the patient to be well rested prior to surgery. The use of both of these agents should be avoided in children under 10 years of age or in patients with liver disease.

CHLORAL HYDRATE

Chloral hydrate is a safe, well tolerated sedative that is useful in children and the elderly. It seldom induces excitement or postsedative "hangover." One major side effect is gastric irritation. This can induce nausea and vomiting and can be avoided by taking the medication on a full stomach or diluting the liquid preparation with milk or water. It is better tolerated if administered in capsule form. It is available as a syrup (500 mg/10 ml and 1 g/10 ml), which is ideal for children, and as 500 mg capsules. The usual dosage is 20 to 40 mg/kg for children and 0.5 to 1.0 g PO for adults. It should be used with caution in patients with liver, renal, or cardiac disease.

It can produce a short-term increase in the hypoprothrombinemic effect of coumarin.

METHOXYFLURANE

Methoxyflurane (Penthrane) is a volatile liquid with a fruity odor that provides partial anesthesia and analgesia when delivered by the manufacturer's hand-held inhaler (Abbott Laboratories). It is particularly helpful in anesthetization of large areas of the head or neck as well as in scalp reduction surgery, hair transplantation, and dermabrasion. Usually, 2 to 3 ml of Penthrane are placed in the inhaler, through which the patient breathes intermittently until becoming lightheaded. The inhaler is refilled every 10 to 15 minutes until the desired degree of analgesia is achieved or until the maximum dose for one sitting (15 ml) is reached.

Methoxyflurane is usually well tolerated and offers a high margin of safety, as continuous dosing requires activity by the patient. Dose-related nephrotoxicity secondary to the metabolites that are formed, fluoride and oxalic acid, has been reported when this agent is used for prolonged periods as a general anesthetic. However, we have not seen this side effect when methoxyflurane is used with the inhaler. Penthrane should not be used in patients with renal dysfunction or hepatic disease or in those taking tetracycline. Since anesthesia with this agent can produce loss of the gag reflex, patients should be non per os (NPO). It should not be administered for more than 4 hours at one sitting. Since it is exhaled by the patient, adequate ventilation is important.

ANTIHISTAMINES

Hydroxyzine (Vistaril) works synergistically with Demerol to provide preoperative sedation. In addition, it has antiemetic properties. It is the preferred sedative for patients with a history of asthma or allergies. Preoperative administration should be parenteral at doses of 25 to 50 mg IM in adults and 1 mg/kg IM in children.

Promethazine (Phenergan) is an antihistamine that is used in a similar manner as hydroxyzine.

NARCOTICS

Meperidine (Demerol) has sedative and analgesic properties and is the drug of choice when more complex procedures, especially on the head and neck, are being performed. The drug produces dryness of the mouth, flushing of the face, sweating, pupillary constriction, euphoria, dizziness, and constipation. It can induce emesis, and is therefore often used in combination with hydroxyzine. When used preoperatively, it must be given parenterally. The usual adult dosage is 50 to 150 mg IM or SQ 20 to 30 minutes before beginning anesthesia. An intravenous set-up and naloxone should always be readily available when Demerol is used, since respiratory depression can occur. Narcotics should be avoided in patients with asthma or other respiratory disease. The pediatric dosage is 1 to 2 mg/kg.

Naloxone (Narcan) should be readily available whenever narcotics are used parenterally. It rapidly reverses the actions of narcotics. It must be given intravenously (0.4 mg) and repeated every 20 minutes because of its short half-life.

MUSIC

The induction of local anesthesia can be accomplished more comfortably by distracting the patient with music or conversation. A very effective method of delivering music to the patient is by using a portable radio or cassette player to which headphones can be attached. This allows patients a choice in what they wish to listen to without disturbing the staff.

RECOMMENDATION

Although the agents listed above may be effective individually, preoperative sedation for larger procedures usually requires the use of a combination of agents. We have found the following regimen helpful:

Diazepam 5 to 10 mg PO or sublingually 30 to 60 minutes before surgery
Meperidine 50 to 150 mg and hydroxyzine 25 to 50 mg IM 20 minutes before
    surgery

9

Clinical Application of Local Anesthesia

There are various methods by which local anesthesia of the skin can be induced. Classified by the application site, they include topical, local infiltration, field block, and peripheral nerve blockade. This chapter's discussion is limited to the uses of these methods in dermatologic surgery.

SAFETY CONSIDERATIONS

Injection of local anesthesia must be considered an invasive procedure. Therefore, it is vital to adhere to the "Universal Guidelines for Protection" as developed by the Centers for Disease Control (CDC). Gloves must be worn. It is recommended to wear protective eyewear, if glasses are not normally worn, to protect against possible spray. Some practitioners advocate masks as well.

The most common cause of surgical injury and healthcare-related human immunodeficiency virus (HIV) infection is needle stick injury. Used needles should not be routinely recapped. Rather, they are best disposed of *by the user* in appropriate, wide-mouthed, puncture-proof containers (Fig. 9-1).

There are instances when recapping needles is necessary. Methods exist that are relatively safe. The first is to lay the needle cap on the surgical tray and advance the needle into the cap without an opposing hand holding the cap (Fig. 9-2). Once the needle is inside the cap, the cap can be safely tightened without risk of puncture. A second method is to place the cap into the bottom of an overturned paper cup (Fig. 9-3) or a piece of 2 inch by 4 inch lumber with appropriately drilled holes. In this position the needle can be safely inserted into the cap.

TOPICAL ANESTHESIA

The use of topical anesthetics on nonmucosal surfaces is limited by relatively poor penetration by the agents presently available. Application times of 1 hour or more under occlusion are necessary to produce anesthesia to the

41

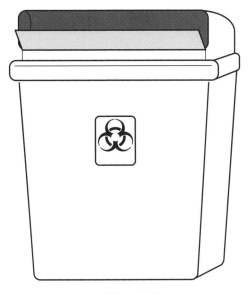

Figure 9-1

level of the papillary dermis. However topical anesthesia of mucosal surfaces is possible due to the relative lack of stratum corneum. In such areas, lidocaine jelly or ointment is the anesthetic of choice. The anesthetic is usually placed on gauze or a cotton ball and held against the mucosal surface. Anesthesia is achievable in 15 minutes or less and is sufficient to allow performance of superficial shave biopsies. In addition, topical anesthesia of

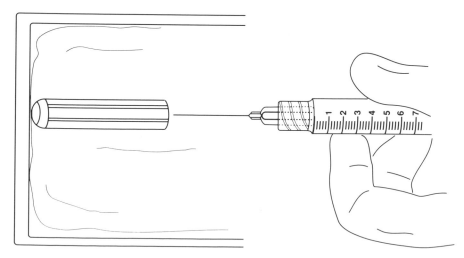

Figure 9-2

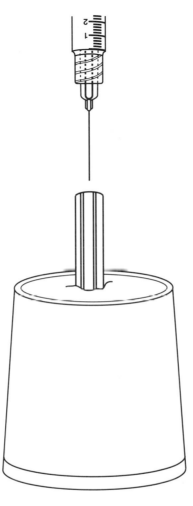

Figure 9-3

the mucosal surface will permit the painless introduction of a needle for providing more extensive anesthesia. This is particularly helpful when it is desired to use the mucosal approach to block branches of the trigeminal nerve. Anesthesia of the conjunctival surface with Ophthane can facilitate the introduction of a needle to anesthetize an eyelid. Cryoanesthesia is discussed in Chapter 7.

INFILTRATION ANESTHESIA

Infiltration anesthesia is defined as the direct placement of a local anesthetic at the nerve endings located in the dermis or subcutaneous fat. An intradermal injection of a local anesthetic produces almost immediate

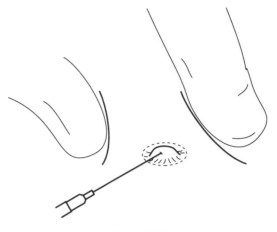

Figure 9-4

anesthesia, the duration of which is prolonged due to better localization. Injection of the anesthetic into the subcutaneous plane is usually less painful than intradermal injection since the former tissue is more distensible. However, the onset of anesthesia is slower and the duration is shorter because subcutaneous diffusion and absorption are more rapid (Figs. 9-4 and 9-5).

A potential problem with infiltration anesthesia is distortion of the operative site (Fig. 9-6). Tissue distortion can be minimized by injecting smaller amounts of anesthesia and by massaging the area after injection. Drawing out

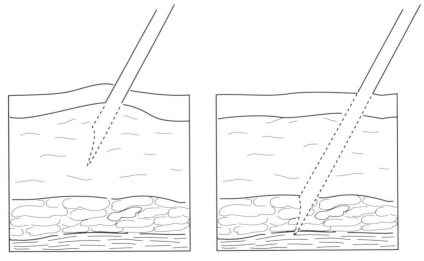

INTRADERMAL   SUBCUTANEOUS

Figure 9-5

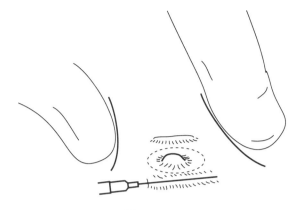

Figure 9-6

the surgical lines before injection helps the surgeon maintain proper orientation should tissue distortion occur. This distention also can be an advantage in performing punch biopsies. The increased tissue turgor will decrease the distorting effects of pressure on the tissue by the punch tool and improve sample quality.

Local anesthetics injected directly into an inflamed or infected area will often fail to produce satisfactory anesthesia. This is due in part to the lower tissue pH that often accompanies acute inflammation. In this situation it is better to perform a field block.

FIELD BLOCKS

Field or ring blocks are variations of infiltration anesthesia. With this technique the actual surgical site is not directly injected. Rather, the anesthetic infiltrates circumferentially around the site, blocking nerve impulses from leaving the area. Ring or field blocks are particularly useful when distortion of the surgical field by direct infiltration is undesirable (such as when anesthetizing cysts, in which injection into the cyst may result in rupture). In skin cancer surgery, field blocks prevent possible implantation of cancer cells beyond the surgical margin. Field blocks are also helpful in limiting the amount of anesthesia required to anesthetize an area. This is particularly important when a large area needs to be anesthetized, such as the scalp in a hair transplant procedure or the trunk when a large excision is planned. The key to success in performing a field block is injecting the anesthetic in both superficial and deep planes (Fig. 9-7).

Scalp Block

Scalp block is a field block that is particularly helpful when large-area procedures are planned on the scalp, such as hair transplantation or scalp reduction.

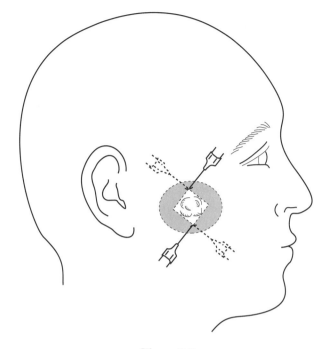

Figure 9-7

Anatomy

The scalp is solely innervated by nerves originating from the periphery. The nerves pass through from under the fascia to lie in a subcutaneous plane on a line encircling the head, drawn above the ear, and passing through the occiput and mid-forehead.

The forehead and anterior scalp are innervated by branches of the ophthalmic division of the trigeminal nerve, which is made up of branches of both the supraorbital and supratrochlear nerves and of the zygomaticotemporal nerve, which originates from the second division of the trigeminal nerve. The temporal region of the scalp is innervated by branches from the second (maxillary) and third (mandibular) divisions of the trigeminal nerve. The occipital and parietal regions are supplied by the greater and lesser occipital nerves originating from the cervical plexus (Fig. 9-8).

Technique

The scalp can be readily anesthetized with a ring block. Any portion of the scalp can be numbed by varying the size of the ring block. The following is a method of anesthetizing the entire scalp (Fig. 9-9).

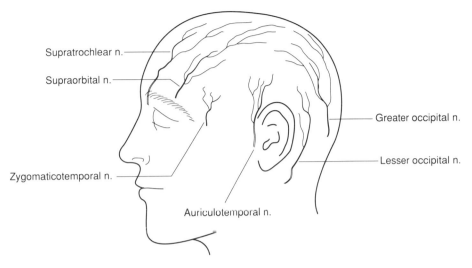

Figure 9-8

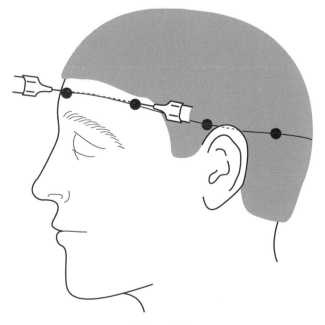

Figure 9-9

Step 1. The temporal arteries are located by palpation relative to the planned ring of anesthesia. It is important to avoid lacerating these vessels.

Step 2. Starting at the mid-forehead and using a 30 gauge needle on a 10 cc syringe, small wheals of anesthesia are made at 2 inch intervals along a ring connecting with the occiput and passing through the level of the superior auricular sulcus.

Step 3. Using a 1.5 or 3.5 inch 25 gauge needle, local anesthetic is injected first subcutaneously and then subfascially, below the galea, between the wheals, "connecting the dots."

Step 4. The temporal fossa must be carefully infiltrated to the temporal bone to secure complete anesthesia, because of the increased muscle mass in the area.

Step 5. Approximately 20 to 30 ml of local anesthetic may be necessary to complete the block. Anesthesia of the scalp is expected within 10 to 15 minutes.

Use of epinephrine with the anesthetic will partially reduce bleeding, inasmuch as the arteries tend to follow the same radial direction as the nerves. However, it is recommended that additional infiltration be carried out along the planned incision lines once the scalp block has taken effect.

Partial failure of the scalp block is high and is often due to inadequate anesthesia at the subfascial plane. For this reason the block should always be tested before beginning surgery.

Several large vessels supply the scalp. Particular care is necessary when injecting into the region of the temporal artery, in order to avoid laceration and hematoma formation. If an artery is punctured, pressure should be held for 20 minutes.

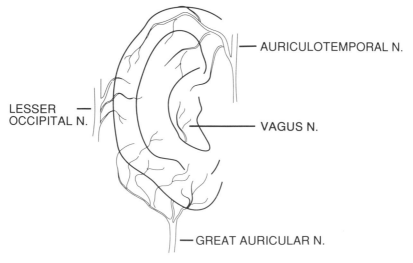

Figure 9-10

Swelling of the eyelids is possible if an excessive amount of anesthesia is injected.

An occasional side effect from extensive surgery of the scalp is postoperative nausea, which can last up to 24 hours. It occurs particularly if the galea is disturbed. This side effect usually responds well to the use of Compazine (prochlorperazine) or Phenergan (promethazine) suppositories (25 mg every 12 hours).

Ear Block

Ear block is a field block that provides anesthesia to the entire ear, except for the concha and external auditory canal.

Anatomy

Sensory innervation of the auricle runs superficially at its external attachment with the head and permits the use of a ring block to anesthetize the ear (Fig. 9-10). The auricle is composed of these three parts:

1. The auriculotemporal nerve, a branch of the third branch of the trigeminal nerve, providing innervation to the anterior one-half of the ear.
2. The great auricular and lesser occipital nerves, branches of the cervical plexus, supplying the posterior half of the ear.
3. The auricular branch of the vagus, which innervates the concha and ear canal. The facial and glossopharyngeal nerves may also supply the concha and ear canal.

Technique

Step 1. A 30 gauge, 1 inch needle on a 10 cc syringe is used.

Step 2. The needle is inserted at the base of the ear, under the lobe, where it attaches with the head. Anesthesia is injected while advancing the needle in a subcutaneous plane to a point just anterior to the tragus (Fig. 9-11).

Step 3. The needle is withdrawn to the insertion point without exiting. It is then redirected and advanced superiorly along the posterior auricular sulcus while injecting anesthesia.

Step 4. The needle is withdrawn and inserted into the preauricular skin at the anterior aspect of the superior auricular sulcus. Anesthesia is injected as the needle is advanced inferiorly towards the tragus. Care must be taken to avoid puncture of the superficial temporal artery.

Step 5. The needle is withdrawn to the point of insertion without exiting. It is redirected posteriorly and advanced along the superior sulcus while injecting anesthetic.

Step 6. The needle is reinserted along the mid-posterior auricular sulcus and

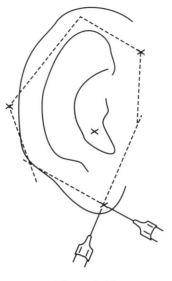

Figure 9-11

directed inferiorly along the posterior sulcus, toward the lobe. It is then withdrawn to the point of insertion and redirected superiorly along the posterior sulcus to complete the ring block.

Step 7. If anesthesia of the concha and ear canal is desired, additional anesthetic will need to be administered by local infiltration.

In patients with arteriolar insufficiency, the use of epinephrine can cause necrosis.

If the temporal artery is accidentally punctured, pressure should be held over the site for 20 minutes.

Nose Block

The nose is a particularly sensitive region on the face to anesthetize by direct infiltration. When a procedure of some size (larger than a biopsy) is planned for the nose, particularly on the nasal tip or alae, a nose block is usually less painful for the patient than local infiltration. A nose block is a ring of anesthesia that blocks the nerves leading to the nasal dorsum, tip, and ala.

Anatomy

The nose is innervated by the ophthalmic and maxillary branches of the trigeminal nerve. At the point where the nasal bone joins with the cartilaginous portion of the nose, the external nasal nerve, a branch of the ophthalmic nerve, exits to innervate the inferior dorsum and nasal tip. The infratrochlear nerve supplies sensory branches to the nasal root and superior nasal dorsum. Terminal branches of the infraorbital nerve run in an inferior and medial

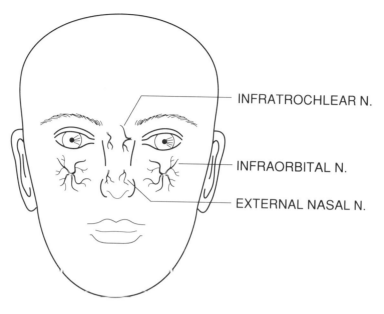

INFRATROCHLEAR N.

INFRAORBITAL N.

EXTERNAL NASAL N.

Figure 9-12

direction to supply sensory innervation to the lateral nasal alae, lateral side-walls, and columella (Fig. 9-12).

Technique

Step 1. The patient lies in a supine position while the anesthetist stands at the head of the bed. A 1 inch, 30 gauge needle on a 10 cc syringe is used.

Step 2. The needle is introduced into the loose skin overlying the root of the nose and a small wheal of anesthetic solution is placed there (Fig. 9-13).

Step 3. The needle is directed in an inferolateral direction, injecting anesthetic solution along the medial canthus to the sidewall of the nose and nasofacial sulcus toward the nasal labial folds bilaterally. It is important to inject both superficially and deeply, (to the bone), in order to get all branches from the infraorbital nerve. Approximately 2 to 4 ml of anesthetic solution is required for each side.

Step 4. The needle is withdrawn to the insertion point, redirected and advanced inferolaterally along the opposite nasal sidewall.

Step 5. The needle is inserted at the lateral ala, just inferior to the superior nasolabial fold. It is advanced superiorly along the nasofacial junction to join the inferior extent of the superior side wall injection (Step 3).

Step 6. The needle is withdrawn to the insertion point and redirected medially along the upper lip just below the nasal sill to the superior philtrum. This anesthetizes the columella.

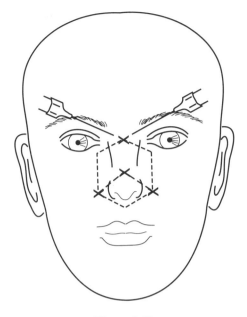

Figure 9-13

Step 7. Steps 5 and 6 are repeated on the opposite side.

Step 8. The needle is inserted in the midnasal dorsum at the joining of the bony and cartilaginous nose. It is then advanced laterally just below this junction toward the inferior nasofacial junction bilaterally. This anesthetizes the external nasal nerves, which supply the nasal tip and medial alae.

An alternative method to injecting along the sidewalls of the nose is performing bilateral infraorbital blocks. The first method is usually preferred, since the latter also anesthetizes the lower eyelids, upper lip, and medial cheeks.

Once a ring block is achieved it is often desirable to infiltrate locally the area to be incised with lidocaine with epinephrine to minimize bleeding.

Occasionally, the inferior aspect of the nasal tip is not anesthetized with the nose block. This is a failure to anesthetize the branch of the infraorbital nerve that supplies the columella. If this occurs, one can infiltrate locally once the rest of the block has taken hold.

PERIPHERAL NERVE BLOCKS

Peripheral nerve blocks inhibit nerve impulse conduction along the nerve trunk rather than suppress the activity at the terminal nerve endings. They have the advantage of anesthetizing a large area while using a relatively small amount of anesthetic. This avoids distortion of the surgical site and results in less patient discomfort, compared with local infiltration.

With peripheral nerve blocks, the local anesthetic is injected subcutaneously. For this reason the onset of anesthesia is delayed from 3 to 10 minutes after injection and the duration is shorter due to more rapid absorption. Although the use of epinephrine can prolong the duration of anesthesia, it usually has minimal effect in decreasing bleeding at the operative site. If vasoconstriction at the operative site is desirable, additional anesthetic with epinephrine will need to be infiltrated locally after the onset of the peripheral nerve blockade.

Since adequate diffusion of the anesthetic is necessary to ensure a successful nerve block, it is advantageous to use the local anesthetic at a higher concentration. The success rate for nerve blocks is increased by using 2 percent lidocaine instead of 1 percent lidocaine.

The duration of a peripheral nerve block can be prolonged by injection of a long-acting agent such as bupivacaine. This can be added after a lidocaine block has taken effect or can be injected simultaneously with 2 percent lidocaine.

Nerve blocks are generally more difficult to perform. Although anatomic landmarks are helpful in locating nerves, individual variation occurs, which must be compensated for when performing this procedure.

Risks of Peripheral Nerve Blocks

When performing peripheral nerve blocks, knowledge of the local anatomy in the area to be injected is particularly important. Potential risks of nerve blocks are discussed below.

Laceration of Nerves with the Needle Point

Laceration of nerves with the needle point can result in long-term or permanent anesthesia in the area supplied by the nerve, which can be prevented in part by avoiding the elicitation of paresthesias during needle placement. *Paresthesias* are shooting or sharp stinging sensations that the patient experiences when a nerve is poked with a needle. These sensations are felt distally in the area supplied by the sensory nerve. Paresthesias indicate that the needle is in the immediate vicinity of the nerve trunk to be anesthetized. Although some believe that one should always try to elicit paresthesias in order to ensure proper placement of the needle, this practice runs the risk of nerve damage. Proper training in the delivery of local anesthesia combined with a knowledge of the local anatomy eliminates the need to elicit paresthesias routinely. If paresthesias are elicited, one should always withdraw the needle 1 to 2 mm until the paresthesias are no longer felt. The risk of nerve damage when performing nerve blocks on the face may be avoided by not attempting to enter the foramina through which the nerves exit.

Intravascular Injection

Blood vessels routinely run with nerves in most areas; therefore, there is always the potential of intravascular injection when performing nerve blocks. Intravascular injection runs the risk of acute toxicity from the local anesthetic and epinephrine. This complication may be avoided by aspirating with the syringe before injecting the local anesthetic. However, the aspiration of blood through a 30 gauge needle is unreliable. For this reason, when performing nerve blocks in areas where intravascular injection is a possibility, it is not unreasonable to use a 25 gauge needle, even though it may produce more pain.

Patients should be observed for several minutes after a nerve block is performed, since reactions to the intravascular injection of local anesthetics can be life-threatening and therefore require immediate action. If adverse signs or symptoms appear at any time during the injection, it should be discontinued.

Hematoma

Even if intravascular injection is avoided, there is always a risk of hematoma formation as a result of vessel laceration. This complication may take up to 2 days to become noticeable. It may be avoided by placing firm pressure over the site of injection for 5 minutes. If bleeding is noted, immediate application of ice and pressure will minimize the size of a hematoma. Treatment with warm soaks will aid in the absorption of a hematoma after it has stabilized in 2 to 3 days.

Paralysis

Paralysis is often temporary and is often due to peripheral blockade of the nerves involved with motor function. The patient should be informed preoperatively of the possibility of this complication. Paralysis lasts approximately 1 to 2 hours and is related to the duration of the anesthetic used. Patients should be kept in the office until reversal occurs or should be called later in the day in order to ascertain that motor function has returned (Fig. 9-14).

Needle Breakage

Another potential local complication of peripheral nerve blocks is the breakage of the needle, which can occur if the needle contacts bone or if an attempt is made to change the direction of the needle without first withdrawing it to a more superficial plane. This is particularly likely to happen when using long, thin needles such as a 3.5 inch, 25 gauge needle or a 1 inch, 30 gauge needle.

Infection

A nerve block should be considered an invasive procedure. Infection with abscess formation can result if the skin is not cleansed properly before performing this procedure. Cleansing the skin surface with alcohol is adequate in otherwise clean or noninfected areas.

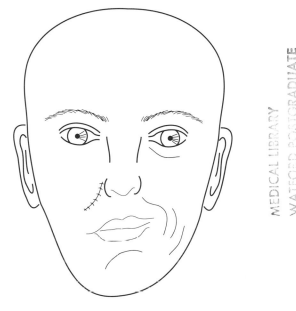

Figure 9-14

Further Considerations

The most commonly employed nerve blocks in dermatologic surgery involve the facial cutaneous branches of the trigeminal nerve. These nerves exit the skull through foramina, which maintain a relatively fixed position from patient to patient. The supraorbital nerve, the infraorbital nerve, and the mental nerve exit-points are vertically oriented along the midpupillary line (Figs. 9-15 and 9-16). This allows the physician to readily locate them and reproducibly perform a blockade.

An important point to keep in mind when performing peripheral nerve blocks is that the nerve supply to the skin varies from patient to patient. Thus, it is necessary to check the extent of anesthesia by light needle taps just before surgery.

Supraorbital and Supratrochlear Block

Supraorbital and supratrochlear nerve blocks provide anesthesia to the entire forehead and frontal scalp.

Anatomy

Supraorbital and supratrochlear nerves are terminal branches of the first division of the trigeminal nerve. The supraorbital nerve passes out of the skull through the supraorbital foramen, which is located approximately 2.5 cm from the facial midline along the inferior edge of the supraorbital ridge. The

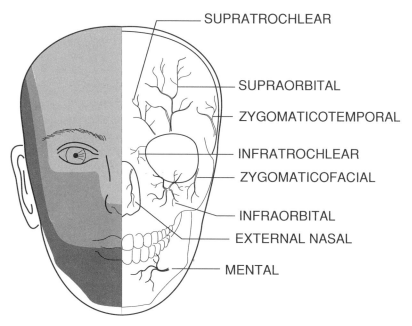

Figure 9-15A

SENSORY PATTERN OF MAJOR TRIGEMINAL NERVE BRANCHES

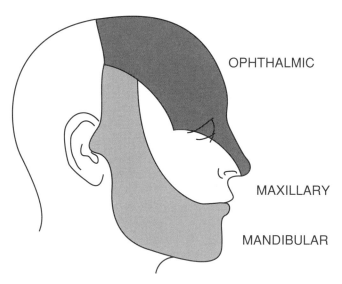

Figure 9-15B

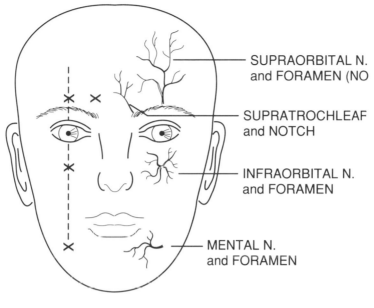

Figure 9-16

supratrochlear nerve issues out of the upper medial corner of the orbit, in the supratrochlear notch, palpable approximately 1.5 cm medial to the supraorbital foramen (Fig. 9-17).

Technique

Step 1. With a gloved finger, locate the supraorbital ridge. Palpate for the supraorbital foramen, which is located approximately 2.5 cm lateral to the midline, along the midpupillary line.

Step 2. After cleansing the skin, a skin wheal is raised above the supraorbital notch, through which the needle is inserted and advanced to bone. Entering the foramen should not be attempted.

Step 3. One to 3 ml of anesthetic is deposited below the level of the inferior frontalis muscle outside the foramen. Parathesias of the supraorbital nerve are characterized by sharp, spraying electric shock sensation over the lateral forehead.

Step 4. The supratrochlear nerve is blocked by advancing the needle medially 1.5 cm and injecting 1 to 2 ml of anesthetic solution at the junction of the medial border of the supraorbital ridge with the root of the nose (Fig. 9-18). Paresthesias may be felt over the medial aspect of the forehead.

An alternative method of blocking the supraorbital and supratrochlear nerves is raising a wheal over the root of the nose and then infiltrating the skin

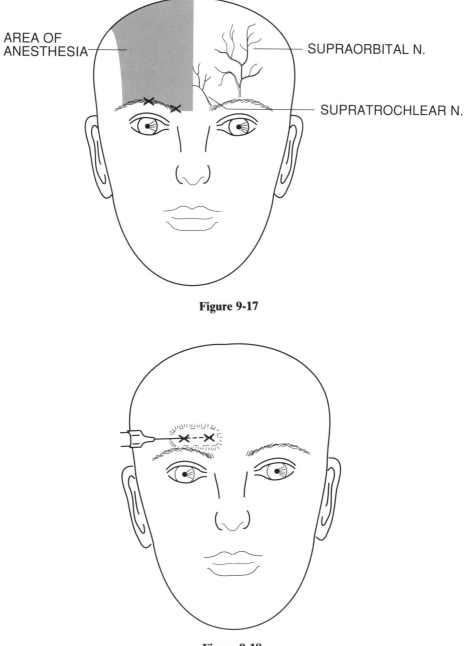

AREA OF
ANESTHESIA

SUPRAORBITAL N.

SUPRATROCHLEAR N.

Figure 9-17

Figure 9-18

along the entire eyebrow. No more than 6 ml should be injected for each side, and 2 to 4 ml are usually sufficient.

Either injection of large quantities of anesthetic solution or hemorrhage can result in swelling of the upper eyelid and, at times, of the lower eyelid. This can interfere with proper lid function. Swelling secondary to excessive local anesthetic will subside in approximately 1 hour. This swelling can be prevented by limiting the amount injected to no more than 2 to 4 ml.

Swelling secondary to hemorrhage will produce discoloration and will persist for 2 to 7 days. This complication can be avoided by applying firm pressure along the supraorbital ridge for several minutes after execution of the block.

Infraorbital Nerve Block

Infraorbital nerve block provides anesthesia to the lower eyelid, medial cheek, side of nose, and upper lip (including mucosal surface).

Anatomy

The infraorbital nerve, a branch of the second division of the trigeminal nerve, emerges from the infraorbital foramen and divides into four branches: inferior palpebral, internal nasal, external nasal, and superior labial. The infraorbital canal lies approximately 2.5 cm lateral to the midline, along the midpupillary line, and just lateral to the frontal process of the maxillary bone, about 1 cm below the infraorbital rim (Fig. 9-19).

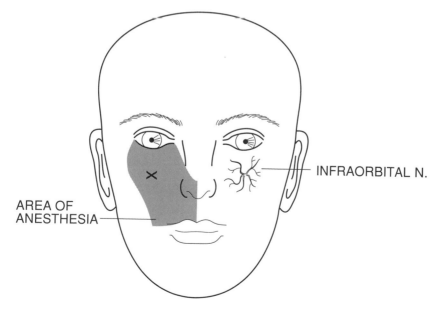

Figure 9-19

Technique

Infraorbital nerve block can be performed using either an external or intraoral approach.

Step 1. *Intraoral and external approaches.* The infraorbital foramen is palpated along the inferior margin of the infraorbital ridge, approximately 2.5 cm from the midline and 1 cm below it.

Step 2. *External approach.* Using a 30 gauge needle on a 5 cc syringe, a wheal is raised 1 cm inferior, and slightly medial, to the foramen.

Step 3. *External approach.* The needle is introduced through the wheal and directed toward the foramen as the index finger of the other hand palpates the foramen. There is usually a 45 degree angle between the skin surface and the shaft of the needle. The needle is advanced in an upward and posterior direction until the point is located in the area of the foramen. Paresthesias of the infraorbital nerve are characterized by sensations in the upper lip, ala of the nose, and upper teeth. If bone is contacted or if parethesia is elicited, the needle should be withdrawn 2 to 3 mm.

Step 4. *External approach.* When the needle is located outside the foramen, 2 to 3 ml of anesthetic is deposited in 0.5 ml portions while changing locations of the needle around the area of the foramen (Fig. 9-20). The enlarging bolus of anesthesia can be palpated, ensuring proper needle placement. It is neither necessary nor advisable to enter the canal.

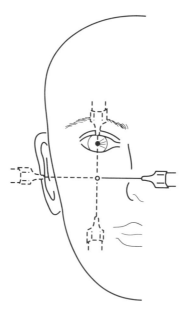

Figure 9-20

Step 2. *Intraoral approach*. While the middle finger of one hand palpates the infraorbital foramen, the thumb and index finger are used to elevate the upper lip.

Step 3. *Intraoral approach*. A 1 inch, 30 gauge needle on a 3 or 5 cc syringe is used. The needle is inserted high into the labial sulcus at the apex of the canine fossa and advanced superiorly towards the foramen until the tip is palpated just outside the foramen (Fig. 9-21). If one has difficulty palpating the needle tip, swelling the tissue by injecting some anesthetic solution can facilitate locating the needle.

Step 4. *Intraoral approach*. When the needle is located just outside the foramen, 2 to 3 ml of anesthetic solution is deposited.

The infraorbital foramen is not always easily palpable; therefore, anesthesia often must be placed based on a knowledge of local anatomy, and especially making use of the midpupillary line.

Introduction of anesthetic solution into the orbit can cause diplopia, pain in the orbit, exophthalmus, blurred vision, or blindness. It may result from misplacement of the needle above the infraorbital rim. It may also be due to the advancement of the needle into the infraorbital foramen and either injecting large volumes of anesthetic solution or puncturing a blood vessel. The latter can be prevented by never introducing the needle into the infraorbital foramen.

Swelling or discoloration of the tissues around the orbit, including swelling of the lower eyelid and, at times, of the upper eyelid, can occur with an

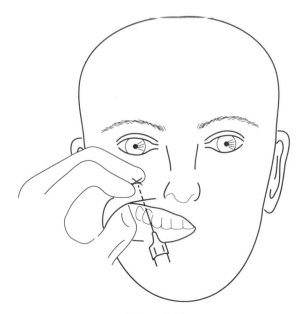

Figure 9-21

infraorbital block. This results either from injecting large quantities of local anesthetic solution or from trauma to the infraorbital vessels. Anesthetic swelling resolves in approximately 1 hour and hemorrhage resolves in 2 to 7 days. Hemorrhage can be prevented by (1) not injecting more than 5 ml of anesthetic solution into the area and (2) applying firm pressure along the infraorbital ridge with the fingers of the free hand during injection.

Using the intraoral approach, infraorbital nerve block can be performed more comfortably for the patient if a topical anesthetic is applied to the mucosal surface before injection.

Mental Nerve Block

Mental nerve block offers a considerably less painful alternative to the direct infiltration of anesthesia when surgery on the lower lip is planned. The mental nerve supplies the lower lip, including the mucosal surface and chin region.

Anatomy

The mental nerve arises from the third division of the trigeminal nerve and exits through the mental foramen (Fig. 9-22). The age of the patient effects the anatomic position of the mental foramen. In the normal adult, the mental foramen is usually located halfway between the upper and lower edges of the mandibular bone, below the apex of the second bicuspid, in the midpupillary line, and approximately 2.5 cm from the midline of the face. In children, the

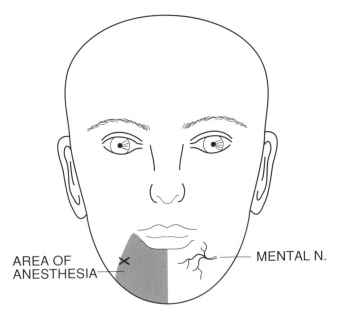

AREA OF
ANESTHESIA

MENTAL N.

Figure 9-22

foramen is frequently located closer to the lower margin of the mandible and is aligned with the first molar. The foramen in older, edentulous patients, due to progressive atrophy of the alveolar ridge, lies closer to the upper border of the mandible.

Technique

There are two methods of performing the mental nerve block: an external and intraoral approach. The advantage of the intraoral method is that the mucosal surface can be readily anesthetized, thereby permitting painless insertion of the needle.

Step 1. *External and Intraoral Approaches.* With the patient's head turned to the side opposite the side to be blocked, the mental foramen is palpated midway between the upper and lower edges of the mandibular bone, along the midpupillary line, which is approximately 2.5 cm from the midline.

Step 2. *External approach.* While palpating the mental foramen, a wheal is raised adjacent to the foramen using a 30 gauge needle on a 5 cc syringe.

Step 3. *External approach.* The needle is advanced through the wheal toward the mental foramen. When the needle is palpated just outside the foramen, 1 to 2 ml of anesthetic solution is injected in 0.5 ml aliquots around the area of the foramen (Fig. 9-23). Paresthesias of the mental

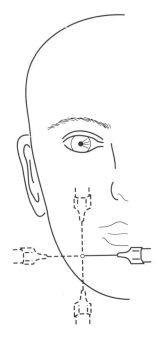

Figure 9-23

nerve are characterized by sensations in the lower lip and occasionally in the anterior lower teeth.

Step 2. *Intraoral approach.* The mental nerve is located inside the lower lip, at the latter's junction with the gum below the second bicuspid. The middle finger of the other hand is used to palpate the foramen while the thumb and forefinger retract the lip. The needle is inserted into the sulcus and advanced only 3 to 4 mm, aiming for the foramen. At the foramen 1 to 2 ml are injected while the middle finger palpates the enlarging bolus of anesthesia (Fig. 9-24).

A bilateral block is necessary if anesthesia of or near the midline skin is needed, due to overlap of the innervation to this region.

Operative procedures that extend to or below the lower margin of the mandible require additional infiltration along the margin of the mandible.

Nerve injury can result, with subsequent numbness of the lower lip, if the needle is inserted into the mental canal. The needle should be withdrawn 2 mm if paresthesias are elicited.

There is a relatively high rate of positive aspirations with this block. It is wise to aspirate before injection and inject the anesthetic slowly.

Mental nerve block can be performed less painfully for the patient by anesthetizing the mucosal surface with a topical anesthetic and using the intraoral approach.

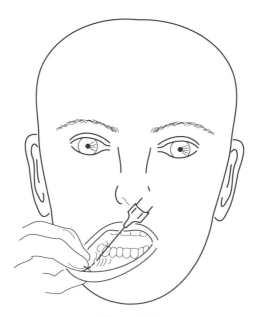

Figure 9-24

Digital Nerve Block

Digital nerve block is a field block that anesthetizes the entire digit. Because there is more subcutaneous space at the proximal finger, it is considerably less painful to inject it than to directly infiltrate the digit distally. This block is particularly useful when nail surgery is planned.

Anatomy

Each digit is innervated by two dorsal nerve branches and two ventral nerve branches as below (Figs. 9-25 and 9-26).

Fingers
    Dorsal surface: radial and ulnar nerves
    Palmar surface: median and ulnar nerves
Toes
    Dorsal surface: peroneal nerve
    Plantar surface: tibial nerve

Occasionally, the dorsal surface of the great toe is in part innervated by the saphenous nerve.

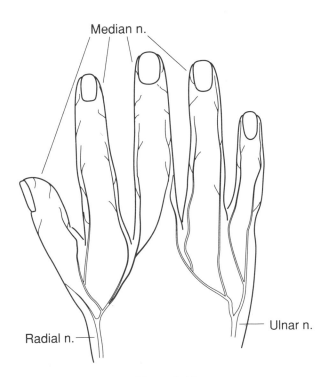

Figure 9-25

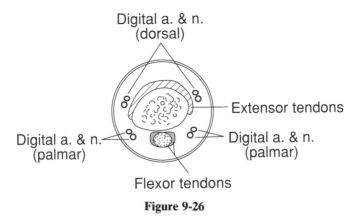

Figure 9-26

Methods

There are two methods by which a digital block is achieved:

1. A ring block around the proximal digit.
2. By directly instilling the anesthetic at the metacarpal/metatarsal heads, before the nerves enter the digit. We usually find the ring block approach more successful, although slightly more risky.

RING BLOCK TECHNIQUE

Step 1. The block is achieved through two injection ports (Fig. 9-27).

Step 2. Using a 1 inch, 30 gauge needle on a 5 or 10 cc syringe, the first injection is made at a dorsolateral margin at the level of the webspace.

Step 3. The needle is advanced across the dorsum, depositing approximately 0.5 to 1.0 ml along both superficial and deep planes.

Step 4. The needle is withdrawn to the entry point without leaving the skin, is then advanced along the lateral surface toward the palmar digital surface, depositing another 0.5 to 1.0 ml, and is then removed.

Step 5. The hand is turned over and the needle is inserted at the palmar medial surface.

Step 6. The needle is then advanced across the palmar surface, withdrawn to the insertion point, and advanced along the medial surface, completing the block.

METACARPAL/METATARSAL HEAD TECHNIQUE

The needle is inserted perpendicular to the skin opposite the heads of the metacarpals/metatarsals. Both dorsal and palmar (plantar) branches are blocked by continuing the injection during the advancement of the needle toward the palm (sole). Approximately 1 to 2 ml of anesthetic solution is deposited on either side of the base of the digit (Fig. 9-28).

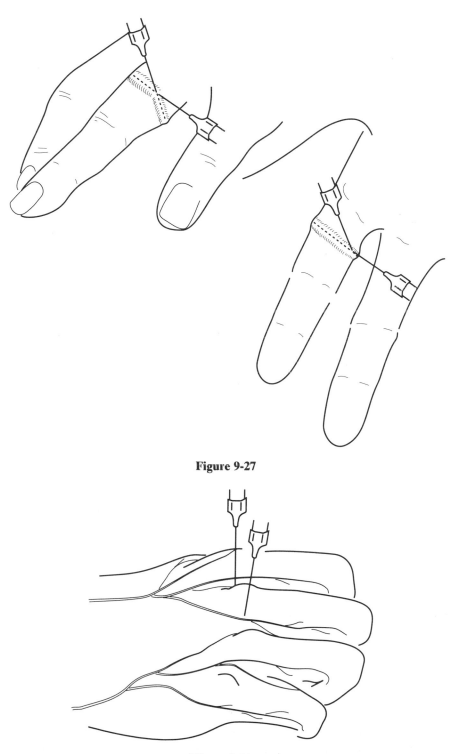

Figure 9-27

Figure 9-28

The metacarpal/metatarsal approach, although safer, is more painful and slower in onset.

Nerve damage is more likely using the ring method. Paresthesia should not be elicited when performing this block.

Intravascular injection in this area is especially dangerous due to the lack of collateral blood vessels and due to the fact that the blood supply consists of terminal branching.

Caution is advised with use of epinephrine. It is generally wise to avoid its use when performing a digital block, although in a healthy, young patient it is probably safe. Its use is contraindicated in an already edematous digit or in the presence of vasospastic diseases. If a prolonged block is desired in these patients, a tourniquet may be used (see below). If one wishes to avoid the use of a tourniquet, a longer-acting anesthetic, such as etidocaine, can be used.

Vascular compression and ischemia can occur when too large a volume of local anesthetic (greater than 8 ml) is used to block the digital nerves. This is particularly true when the block is performed on an already edematous digit or peripheral vascular disease is present.

An unsatisfactory block is usually secondary to failure to infiltrate close to the bone, where the nerves lie. The digital block will occasionally fail if plain lidocaine is used without a tourniquet. Another reason for an unsuccessful block is failure to anesthetize an adequate length of the nerve. These problems can be avoided by using the anesthetic at a higher concentration.

Use of a Tourniquet

Plain lidocaine is rapidly absorbed; therefore, a tourniquet is sometimes helpful to increase the duration of the block. A proper tourniquet should be placed at the base of the digit, proximal to the site on which the ring block was performed. We usually use a one-quarter in penrose drainage tube. A hemostat is used to hold the tourniquet in place around the digit. The tourniquet should be tight enough to stop arterial blood flow; otherwise the digit will become swollen and purple. In an otherwise healthy patient with good circulation, a tourniquet can be left in place for up to 1 hour.

Penis Block

Penis block is considerably less painful than the direct infiltration of anesthesia, especially when surgery on the glans or prepuce is planned. It provides anesthesia distal to the ring of anesthesia.

Anatomy

The innervation of the penis is derived from terminal branches of the pudendal plexus, which form the dorsal nerves of the penis after passing under the symphysis pubis and piercing the suspensory ligament of the penis. They then run along the dorsal surface of the penis, just under the deep fascia

(Buck's fascia), and send off several smaller branches, which pass circumferentially around the penis to supply the lateral and ventral aspects. The base of the penis is supplied by the ilioinguinal nerve and occasionally by a branch of the genitofemoral nerve.

Technique

Step 1. The inferior border of the symphysis pubis, which is located just above the root of the penis, is palpated.

Step 2. A 30 gauge needle on a 10 cc syringe is inserted first through the skin at the 2 o'clock position, relative to the base of the penis, and directed in a caudal direction along the inferior border of the symphysis pubis until a "pop" is felt as the needle pierces the deep fascia of the penis.

Step 3. If aspiration of blood is negative, 10 ml of local anesthetic is deposited. It is important to inject close to the pubic bone in order to block the dorsal nerve before any branching has taken place. If not, sensation may remain intact along the undersurface of the penis.

Step 4. The procedure is repeated on the opposite side, at the 10 o'clock position.

Step 5. Supplemental infiltration both subcutaneously and subfascially at the base along the lateral and ventral surface may be added if the block is not complete in 10 minutes.

An easier, alternative method is to perform a ring block by injecting the anesthetic both subcutaneously and subfascially circumferentially around the penis. Anesthesia is induced distal to this block (Fig. 9-29).

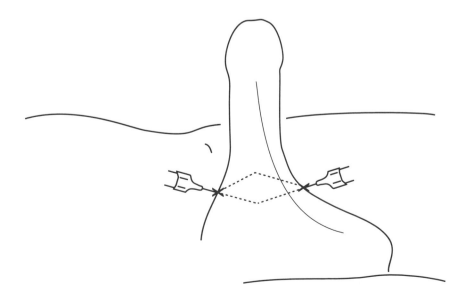

Figure 9-29

The rich vascularization of the penis probably protects it from epinephrine-induced necrosis; however, it is advisable to use plain lidocaine in order to reduce the risk of a possible necrotic incident, especially in patients with occlusive vascular disease. If a longer-duration block is desired, etidocaine should be used.

Caution must be used if a ring block method is chosen to anesthetize the penis. Excessive anesthetic placed around the base of the penis can constrict the blood supply and result in necrosis. No more than 10 ml should be injected around the penis.

Hemorrhage into the shaft of the penis may occur. This can be avoided by using a fine-caliber needle (30 gauge).

Impotency has been occasionally reported after penis block, and is probably related to nerve damage.

Infiltration of the prepuce with large amounts of anesthesia can result in sloughing.

Ankle Blocks

Ankle nerve blocks are more complicated than the other procedures described, but with appropriate knowledge of the anatomy they can be performed with consistency and safety. They are quite valuable when surgery on the plantar surface is planned, as injections into the sole are very painful. If a long-acting local anesthetic is used, excellent postoperative analgesia is possible. A posterior ankle block will anesthetize the sole, while an anterior ankle block will anesthetize the dorsal surface of the foot.

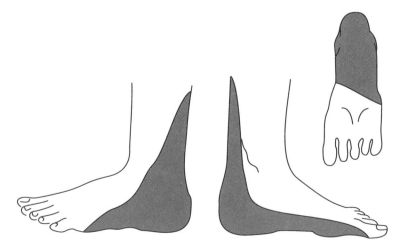

Figure 9-30

Posterior Ankle Block

ANATOMY

The sural nerve runs lateral to the Achilles tendon to innervate the posterior and lateral aspect of the sole (Fig. 9-30). At the level of the lateral malleolus, it is fairly superficial and lies between the Achilles tendon and the lateral malleolus (Fig. 9-31).

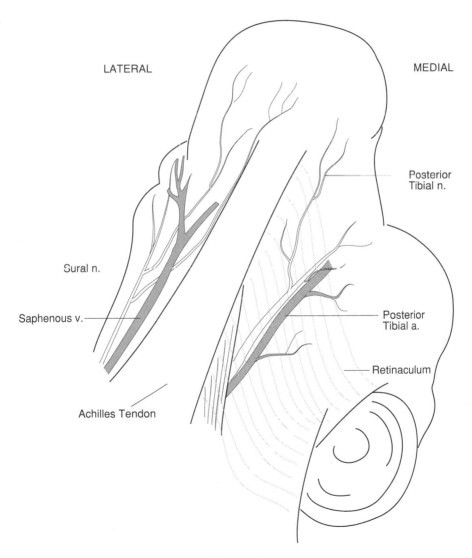

Figure 9-31

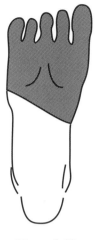

Figure 9-32

The posterior tibial nerve runs medial to the Achilles tendon to innervate the anterior and medial aspect of the sole (Fig. 9-32). At the ankle, the posterior tibial nerve lies posterolaterally to the posterior tibial artery, which is easily palpable just behind the medial malleolus (Fig. 9-31).

TECHNIQUE

Step 1. The patient is placed in a prone position and the ankle is supported on a pillow. To perform a posterior ankle block it is necessary to anesthetize both the sural and posterior tibial nerves.

Step 2. Using a 30 gauge needle on a 10 cc syringe, the sural nerve is blocked by subcutaneous infiltration at the level of the ankle extending from the lateral aspect of the Achilles tendon to the border of the lateral malleolus (Fig. 9-33). Approximately 5 to 8 ml of local anesthetic solution is deposited.

Step 3. The posterior tibial nerve is located by first palpating the posterior tibial artery, which lies just behind the medial malleolus. The nerve is immediately posterior and lateral to the pulsations.

Step 4. If the artery is palpated, the needle should be inserted approximately two fingerbreadths posterior to the medial malleolus and directed posterior and lateral to the pulsations. If paresthesias are elicited, the needle should be withdrawn several millimeters in order to avoid injecting the nerve directly. At this point, 3 to 8 ml of anesthetic solution is deposited in this region (Fig. 9-34).

Step 6. If the artery is not palpable, the needle is inserted just medial to the Achilles tendon at the level of the proximal aspect of the medial malleolus and directed toward the second toe. A 22 gauge spinal

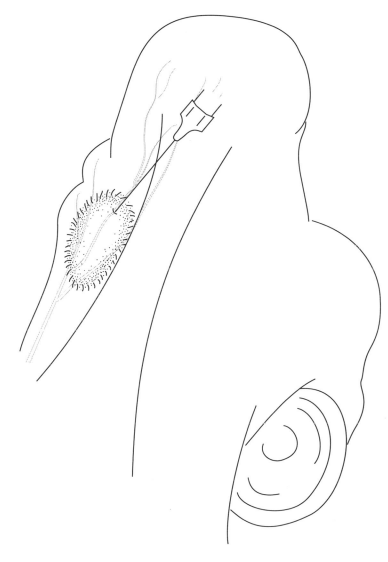

Figure 9-33

needle may be needed. The needle is advanced until paresthesia or bone is encountered. At that point, 5 to 10 ml of anesthetic solution is deposited.

Epinephrine should not be used in patients with ischemic lesions of the foot or advanced diabetes.

It is important to aspirate before injection in order to avoid intravascular injection.

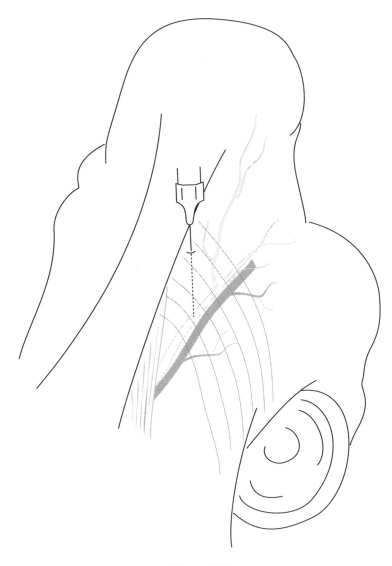

Figure 9-34

Partially effective ankle blocks still allow administration of supplemental local infiltrative anesthesia with less discomfort to the patient at the surgical site.

Allow up to 15 or 20 minutes for the block to take effect.

Anterior Ankle Block

An anterior ankle block provides anesthesia to the dorsum of the foot. To block the entire dorsum of the foot three nerves must be anesthetized; the

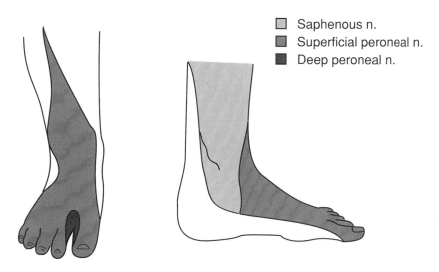

□ Saphenous n.
▨ Superficial peroneal n.
■ Deep peroneal n.

Figure 9-35

superficial peroneal nerve, the deep peroneal nerve, and the saphenous nerve (Fig. 9-35). Since the superficial peroneal nerve innervates a major portion of the dorsum of the foot, it is rarely necessary to block all three nerves.

SUPERFICIAL PERONEAL NERVE BLOCK

Anatomy
The superficial peroneal nerve perforates the fascia on the anterior aspect of the distal two-thirds of the leg and runs subcutaneously down to the dorsum of the foot. It innervates the dorsum of the foot, except for the first webspace (Fig. 9-36).

Technique
Step 1. At the level of the upper part of the lateral malleolus, approximately 5 to 10 ml of anesthetic solution is injected subcutaneously from the anterior border of the tibia to the lateral malleolus (Fig. 9-37).

The block can be enhanced by continuing the subcutaneous infiltration medially to the medial malleolus. This will also anesthetize the saphenous nerve.

To anesthetize the first webspace the deep peroneal nerve needs to be blocked.

SAPHENOUS NERVE BLOCK

Anatomy
The saphenous nerve follows the great saphenous vein to innervate the skin around the medial malleolus (Fig. 9-36).

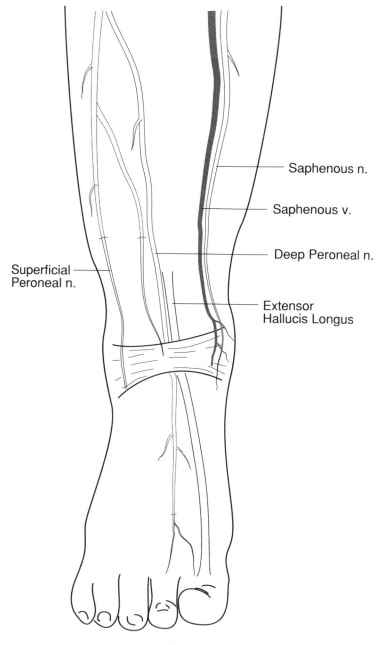

Figure 9-36

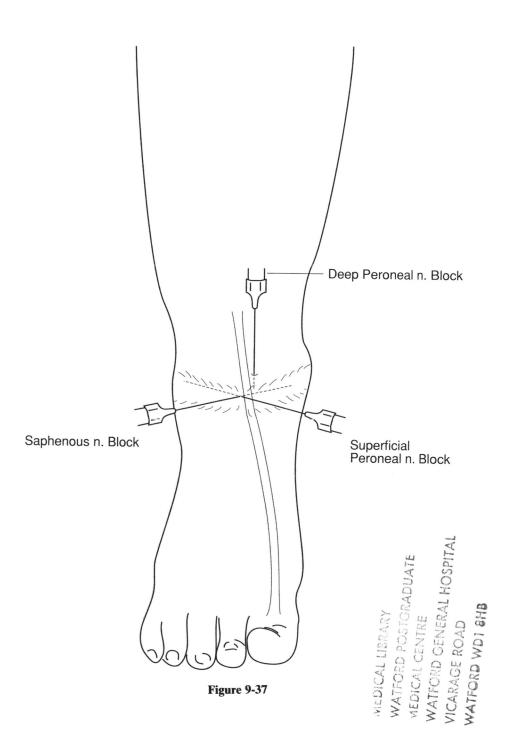

Figure 9-37

Technique

Step 1. The nerve is located just lateral to the vein. The vein can often be visualized by having the leg hang in a dependent position.

Step 2. Approximately 5 to 10 ml of anesthetic solution is deposited subcutaneously around the great saphenous vein, immediately above and just anterior to the medial malleolus (Fig. 9-37).

Care must be taken not to inject local anesthetic solution into the vein. This is particularly a problem in patients with varicose veins.

DEEP PERONEAL NERVE BLOCK

Anatomy

At the level of the malleolus, the peroneal nerve lies deep to the extensor retinaculum with the anterior tibial artery on the anterior tibial surface of the distal end of the tibia, between the tendons of the extensor hallucis longus and tibialis anterior (Fig. 9-36). It innervates the skin of the first webspace (Fig. 9-35).

Technique

Step 1. Tendons of the extensor hallucis longus and tibialis anterior are located by having the patient dorsiflex the foot and toes.

Step 2. Palpation lateral to the extensor hallucis tendon will identify the anterior tibial artery. The nerve lies medial to the extensor hallucis longus tendon and anterior tibial artery. The needle is inserted perpendicular to the skin and medial to the extensor hallucis tendon until bone is felt. Here 5 to 10 ml of anesthetic solution is injected in a fanwise manner in the medial lateral plane, to infiltrate the entire compartment.

Deep peroneal nerve block is rarely needed in dermatology and is only included for the sake of completeness. Local infiltration is generally adequate between the first two toes for anesthesia of this area.

10

Tricks to Make the Delivery of Local Anesthesia Less Painful

The thoughtful use of local anesthesia can greatly improve the patient's experience of the surgical procedure. If improperly performed, the induction of local anesthesia can hurt considerably more than the proverbial mosquito bite. There are three principal sources of pain during the induction of local anesthesia (Fig. 10-1):

1. The needle puncture at the skin surface
2. Tissue irritation by the anesthetic solution
3. Tissue distention by the anesthetic solution

In this chapter we discuss some "tricks" for minimizing pain from each of these three sources.

THE NEEDLE PUNCTURE

Antianxiety Measures

Simply explaining to the patient what is to be expected during the induction of local anesthesia can go a long way in allaying the fears of those who have no prior knowledge of the procedure. In patients who claim extreme anxiety over needle sticks, premedication with diazepam or another antianxiety agent is particularly helpful.

Topical Anesthetic Use on Nonmucosal Surfaces

Pain from the needle puncture can be eliminated entirely by using a topical anesthetic. This is particularly useful in the pediatric population. Unfortunately, nonmucosal surfaces are rather resistant to topical anesthetic

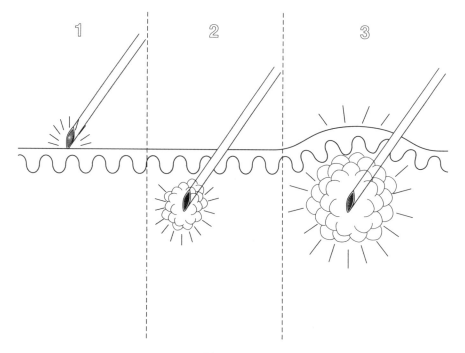

Figure 10-1

agents. Application times under occlusion exceeding 1 hour are necessary to anesthetize the skin surface down to the papillary dermis. Thus, topical anesthesia for this purpose is most practical if it is applied by the patient at home before the planned surgery. Lidocaine jelly or cream in concentrations from 5 percent to 30 percent is presently used and is applied under occlusion at least 2 hours before the appointment. When eutectic mixture of local anesthesia (EMLA) becomes available in the United States it may be the preferred agent for this purpose.

Refrigerant sprays offer an advantage over topical anesthetic agents in that they produce immediate surface anesthesia, thereby permitting painless needle insertion. Overzealous use, however, can produce pain and other side effects (e.g., blistering, hypopigmentation).

Topical Anesthetic Use on Mucosal Surfaces

Mucosal surfaces are much more readily anesthetized with topical anesthetics; application times of less than 15 minutes with 5 percent lidocaine jelly will anesthetize a mucosal surface to pinprick. Thus, if possible, it is preferable to use a mucosal route to anesthetize a skin surface. This is particularly helpful if one wishes to anesthetize the lip. A mucosal approach can also be used to perform an infraorbital or mental nerve block.

The eyelids can be a particularly painful area to anesthetize. Installation of

Ophthane (or another ophthalmic anesthetic solution) into the conjunctival sulcus can anesthetize this surface sufficiently to painlessly introduce a needle for anesthetization of the eyelid.

Smaller-Diameter Needles

Smaller-diameter needles are considerably less painful for the patient. In general, we use a 30 gauge needle for most anesthesia procedures.

Longer Needles

The use of longer needles reduces the number of needle sticks necessary to anesthetize a larger area. For most work, we use a 1 inch, 30 gauge needle. When anesthetizing larger areas, we find a 22 or 25 gauge spinal needle particularly helpful in reducing patient discomfort, because it decreases the necessary number of needle sticks.

Long-Acting Anesthetics

If a fairly long surgical procedure is contemplated, it is desirable to use a long-acting anesthetic in order to reduce the need for repeated injections. These agents do, however, have a fairly long onset of action. For this reason, two agents are usually either injected simultaneously or sequentially, using lidocaine as the second, short-onset agent.

Manipulation of the Skin at the Injection Site

Distracting the patient by slightly pinching or vibrating the skin to be injected may help decrease the perception of pain by the patient. This will also help minimize pain from tissue distention and irritation.

Insertion through an Accentuated Pore

Insertion of the needle through an accentuated pore, particularly, on the face, is less painful (Fig. 10-2).

Careful Insertion Technique

The insertion of the needle should be done slowly and gently with the bevel pointed down. A quick, jabbing approach increases patient discomfort.

Choice of Reinsertion Site

When anesthetizing larger areas of skin, one should reinsert the needle into an area already anesthetized.

Avoidance of Reinjection

Adequate time should be allowed for the anesthetic to work before area is reinjected. There is usually some delay in the onset of anesthesia, unless it is injected close to the surface. Anesthesia can be delayed up to several minutes

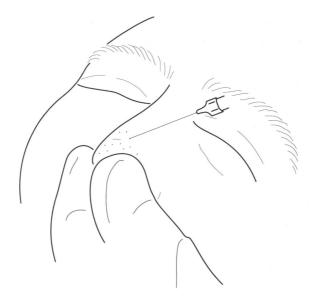

Figure 10-2

when injected in a subcutaneous plane and up to 15 minutes with some nerve blocks. Impatience on the part of the physician can lead to an unnecessary reinjection and additional discomfort for the patient.

TISSUE IRRITATION

Anesthetic solutions are usually prepared at a pH considerably more acidic than tissue pH for preservation of the agents. This difference in pH produces tissue irritation when the anesthetic is injected, which is experienced as a burning sensation. Lidocaine with epinephrine produces considerably more burning than plain lidocaine when injected. The reason for this is due to the difference in pH, as shown here.

	pH
Lidocaine with epinephrine	3.5–4.5
Plain lidocaine	6.5–6.8
Tissue fluid	7.3–7.4

Since tissue irritation from local anesthetics is due in large part to the acidity of the solution, one method of reducing this cause of discomfort is increasing the pH of the anesthetic solution. If epinephrine is needed there are several ways of doing this, including the following:

1. The simplest method is mixing equal parts of plain lidocaine with lidocaine with epinephrine. This will produce a solution that is less painfully injected than unaltered lidocaine with epinephrine.

2. Another method involves starting with plain lidocaine and freshly adding a small amount of concentrated epinephrine from an ampule (0.1 ml epinephrine at 1 : 1,000 to 10 ml of plain lidocaine). This will produce a solution, with a pH identical to plain lidocaine, that is less painfully injected than commercially prepared lidocaine with epinephrine.
3. The third method is neutralizing the commercially prepared lidocaine with epinephrine with sodium bicarbonate. Sodium bicarbonate (8.4 percent solution) is added to lidocaine with epinephrine at a 1 : 10 ratio (1 part bicarbonate to 9 parts anesthetic). This will produce a solution with a pH very close to that of tissue fluid. This method has proved the least painful in injecting lidocaine with epinephrine.

Some practitioners feel that the duration of anesthesia with a buffered solution is somewhat shorter, compared with that of the unaltered product. This may be due to a more rapid absorption of the less charged buffered agents across tissue membranes facilitating "wash out." For this reason, once numbness is achieved, it is recommended that the anesthesia be reinforced with a nonbuffered anesthetic or a long-acting anesthetic if a lengthy procedure is anticipated.

TISSUE DISTENTION

Tissue distention is experienced by the patient as a burning sensation. It is particularly likely to occur when the anesthetic solution is injected into tissue that has a limited ability to expand.

Slow Administration of the Anesthetic

The pain secondary to tissue distention is related in part to the rate at which anesthesia is injected. Rapid injections are associated with greater pain. The anesthetic should be administered slowly, allowing the stretch receptors time to accommodate the new volume of fluid.

Limiting the Amount of Anesthetic Solution

Pain from tissue distention is also related to the volume of fluid injected: the greater volume of fluid injected, the greater the discomfort caused by tissue distention. Thus, it is wise to avoid injecting excessive amounts of anesthetic solution.

Injection into the Subcutaneous Fat

Injection into the subcutaneous fat is always less painful than an intradermal injection close to the skin surface, since fat has a greater ability to expand than does the dermis. However, injection into the fat has a longer onset of action and a shorter duration, whereas intradermal injection has an almost immediate onset of action with a longer duration of action.

Use of Field Blocks

Areas with a tightly bound dermis and little subcutaneous fat, such as the tip of the nose and the nail folds of the digits are particularly uncomfortable areas to inject. In these areas it is often less painful to anesthetize the area with a field block (Ch. 9) rather than with direct infiltration.

Careful Approach to Bone

Bone should always be approached carefully, since periosteum is sensitive to needle sticks.

Proper Direction of Injection

Injection should always begin proximally and advance distally, in the same direction as the innervation. This is particularly helpful on the extremities, where this technique often produces anesthesia distal to the initial injection site, thereby decreasing patient discomfort.

Careful Injection of the Palmar or Plantar Surfaces

Injection into the palmer or plantar surfaces can be quite painful, due to an increased number of nerve endings and an adherent dermis with limited ability to expand. A much less painful approach is first to introduce the anesthetic into the dorsal skin adjacent to the area to be anesthetized. The needle is then advanced toward the plantar or palmar surface. If the site to be injected is in the center of the plantar or palmer surface, a stepwise approach may be necessary. A posterior ankle block (Ch. 9) may obviate the need to inject the plantar surface.

11

Procedure-Oriented Anesthesia

LIP BLOCK

Anesthesia only of the lips is sometimes desirable for minimizing discomfort during lip augmentation with either collagen or fat or if excisional surgery on the lip is planned.

Anatomy

The upper lip receives its innervation from the infraorbital branch of trigeminal nerve. The lower lip is innervated by terminal branches of the mental nerve (see Fig. 9-15).

Technique

Step 1. Anesthesia of the upper lips can be accomplished almost painlessly by using an intraoral approach. The mucosal surface at the labial sulcus and the oral commissures is first anesthetized using 5 percent lidocaine jelly for 10 to 15 minutes.

Step 2. Once the mucosal surface is anesthetized, a 30 gauge needle on a 10 cc syringe is inserted at the commissure and directed first submucosally and then subcutaneously along a line connecting the commissure with the nasal ala. Approximately 1 to 2 ml of anesthetic are deposited (Fig. 11-1).

Step 3. Step 2 is repeated in a similar manner at the other commissure.

Step 4. To anesthetize the lower lip, a wheal is raised at the midpoint of the chin.

Step 5. The needle is inserted through this wheal and directed obliquely toward the corner of the mouth. Two to five ml of anesthetic are injected along the subcutaneous and submucosal plane (Fig. 11-1).

Step 6. The needle is withdrawn and redirected in a similar manner toward the other angle of the mouth.

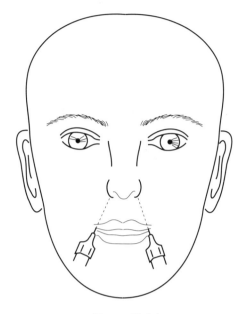

Figure 11-1A

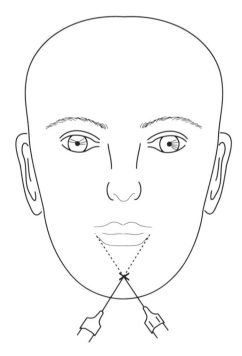

Figure 11-1B

An alternative method of anesthetizing the lower lip is by performing bilateral mental nerve blocks.

Care must be taken not to inject too much anesthetic solution, so as to avoid distorting the lip.

If the upper lip block is unsatisfactory, supplemental injections are made through the mucosal surface along the superior sulcus of the lip.

HAIR TRANSPLANTATION/SCALP REDUCTION

A scalp block is the most efficient way to produce anesthesia of the scalp for hair transplantation or scalp reduction (see Ch. 8). A complete ring block is needed for a scalp reduction. Supplemental injection into proposed incisional lines will aid hemostasis after the block has taken. For hair transplantation, injection need be only around the actual recipient site; along the frontal "U" of the hairline is sufficient for frontal transplants (Fig. 11-2). Since the harvesting of plugs with hair transplantation surgery tends to occur at a site distant from the recipient site, the donor site is usually anesthetized separately with the use of a local infiltration approach. Local infiltration, rather than ring block, aids hemostasis.

DERMABRASION/CHEMICAL PEELS

In dermabrasion or chemical peel, anesthesia of the entire face is sometimes desired. If the freezing technique is used with dermabrasion, often the refrigerant alone is sufficient to produce anesthesia; otherwise a face block becomes necessary.

Anesthesia of the entire face may be most easily accomplished by first performing a trigeminal nerve block. All three branches of the trigeminal nerve (supraorbital/supratrochlear nerve, infraorbital nerve, and mental nerve) need to be blocked (see Ch. 9 and Fig. 9-15). A field block is then performed by carrying a ring of anesthesia from the eyebrows inferiorly along the side of the face (pretragal) and along the jawline (Fig. 11-3). This can be most easily accomplished by first raising superficial wheals at the 2, 3, 5, 7, 9, and 10 o'clock positions using a 1 inch, 30 gauge needle. These points can then be connected with a 25 gauge spinal needle. This will produce anesthesia medial to the ring of anesthesia, except for the dorsum and tip of nose. To anesthetize this area, a dorsal nasal block must be performed.

An alternative method of anesthetizing the lateral two-thirds of the cheek involves inserting the needle anterior to the ear and locally infiltrating the anesthetic through a sequence of injections extending radially from this point.

Pain can be considerable immediately after dermabrasion or chemical peel. This discomfort can be lessened by applying gauze soaked with anesthetic solution to the treated areas. Since the normal skin barriers are disrupted, anesthesia occurs almost instantly. The addition of epinephrine 1 : 100,000 to the anesthetic solution will provide vasoconstriction adequate to stop bleeding after dermabrasion. These steps will make subsequent bandaging easier for the patient.

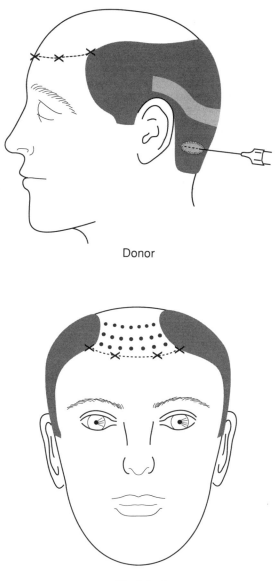

Donor

Recipient

Figure 11-2

BLEPHAROPLASTY

During cosmetic surgery on the eyelids it is important that tissues not be distorted by excessive anesthesia. It is always wise for the surgeon to mark and measure the proposed incision lines before injecting the anesthetic.

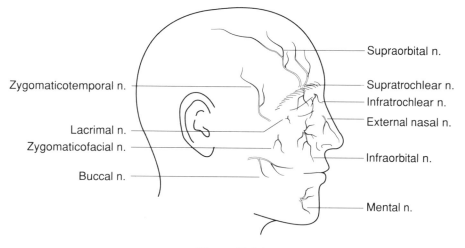

Supraorbital n.

Zygomaticotemporal n.

Supratrochlear n.
Infratrochlear n.
External nasal n.

Lacrimal n.
Zygomaticofacial n.

Infraorbital n.

Buccal n.

Mental n.

Figure 11-3A

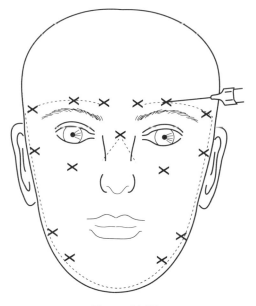

Figure 11-3B

Due to the peripheral innervation of the eyelids by the supraorbital, in-fraorbital, infratrochlear, and lacrimal nerves, anesthesia is possible by using a field block along the orbital rim (Figs. 9-15 and 11-4). This method has the advantage over direct infiltration in that distortion of the eyelids is minimized. Lidocaine 1 percent with epinephrine at 1 : 200,000 is used, and no more than 2 to 3 ml of local anesthetic is needed to anesthetize each upper eyelid. Excessive anesthesia in this area may affect levator function and distort

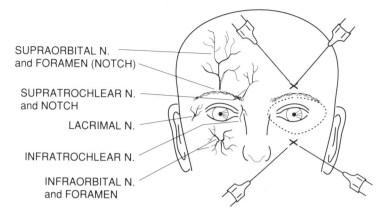

SUPRAORBITAL N. and FORAMEN (NOTCH)

SUPRATROCHLEAR N. and NOTCH

LACRIMAL N.

INFRATROCHLEAR N.

INFRAORBITAL N. and FORAMEN

Figure 11-4

relationships between anatomic planes. A dose of 3 to 5 ml of anesthetic is adequate to anesthetize each lower lid. It is necessary to wait at least 15 to 20 minutes after injection in order to allow adequate dispersion of the anesthetic. The conjunctival surfaces will need to be anesthetized separately using a topical agent.

An alternative method is to locally infiltrate the eyelids with 1 to 2 percent lidocaine and epinephrine containing hyaluronic acid (150 U/30 ml). It is felt that this method offers better dispersion of the anesthetic. The disadvantage of this method is that intraoperative reinforcement with the same anesthetic may be necessary.

The use of a long-acting anesthetic, such as bupivacaine, is probably best avoided during this procedure since orbicularis oculi function can be compromised for a prolonged period, leading to corneal drying.

OTHER EYELID PROCEDURES

Occasionally it is desirable to distort the eyelid with excessive anesthesia. This is particularly the case when one wishes to perform a shave or punch biopsy of the eyelid or carbon dioxide laser procedures. The extra anesthetic fluid not only makes it easier to perform the biopsy, because of the increased turgor of the tissue, but it also provides a safety cushion against injury to the eye.

LIPOSUCTION

It has been demonstrated repeatedly that liposuction using the wet or tumescent technique is vastly superior to the dry technique, which requires general anesthesia. The wet technique uses standard concentrations of lidocaine (0.5 to 1.0 percent) with epinephrine (1 : 100,000) to anesthetize the area to be treated. The tumescent technique differs in that a large amount of very dilute local anesthetic solution is used. The tumescent technique is currently the preferred method for liposuction. Its main advantage over the wet technique is that blood levels of lidocaine are greatly reduced. By using the tumescent technique more than twice the maximal recommended dose for lidocaine can be used. The formula for this dilute anesthetic solution is as follows (see Klein, Suggested Readings):

500 mg lidocaine	50 ml 1% plain lidocaine
1 mg epinephrine	1 ml 1 : 1,000 epinephrine
12.5 mEq sodium bicarbonate	12.5 ml sodium bicarbonate (1 mEq/ml)
9 g NaCl	1 liter 0.9% NaCl in standard IV bag

This formula results in a solution containing 0.05 percent lidocaine, epinephrine 1 : 1,000,000, and 12.5 mEq/l sodium bicarbonate in 0.84 percent NaCl. The anesthesia that is produced in 15 to 20 minutes is sufficient to obviate the need for intravenous sedation. Some recommend adding 1,500 units of hyaluronic acid to this formula in order to facilitate diffusion. However, this is probably unnecessary using the tumescent technique since wide diffusion is ensured. There is also concern that use of hyaluronic acid will increase the rate of absorption into the circulation and decrease the duration of anesthesia.

Installation of the dilute anesthetic solution can be facilitated by the use of the McGhan refilling tissue expander syringe (Fig. 11-5). This syringe can be connected to an intravenous bag containing the dilute anesthetic solution. The syringe rapidly refills itself after each injection due to a spring device and a one-way valve, which greatly speeds the rate at which the anesthetic can be injected. Use of a 3 inch, 22 gauge spinal needle reduces the number of needle sticks necessary to anesthetize an area.

One of the major concerns about this technique is that a large amount of

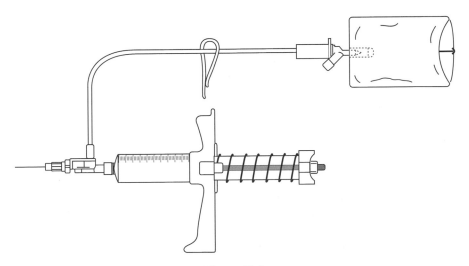

Figure 11-5

lidocaine is injected at one sitting. The actual blood levels after this procedure however, are much lower than expected (<1 µg/ml). There are several possible reasons for this. First, some of the anesthetic solution is aspirated during the procedure. Second, adipose tissue is relatively avascular, thus absorption into the blood is reduced. Third, since a lower concentration of lidocaine is used, the concentration gradient causing it to go into the circulation is less. Fourth, as lidocaine is partially lipid-soluble, some of the remaining anesthetic is probably absorbed into the fat that stays behind. Still, many voice concern over potential toxicity from using large amounts of lidocaine. For this reason, some physicians advocate the use of preoperative diazepam (10 mg) to raise the seizure threshold to lidocaine.

MOHS SURGERY

Mohs micrographic surgery is often a lengthy procedure requiring multiple stages. Therefore, the use of a longer-acting local anesthetic may be beneficial. The use of etidocaine or bupivacaine will offer prolonged anesthesia, especially if used in combination with a nerve block. Anesthesia for the initial stage may be obtained with lidocaine. At the end of the stage, an injection of a long-acting agent may ensure anesthesia if a subsequent stage or repair is needed.

Nerve blocks, especially of the nose, ear, and branches of the trigeminal nerve, are useful when performing Mohs surgery. Nerve blocks offer a less painful alternative to direct infiltration of anesthesia in these areas.

The incorporation of a local anesthetic with the gauze used to cover the Mohs defect in between stages can help minimize discomfort to the patient. Since systemic absorption occurs, it is important to monitor the amount of anesthetic used, in order to avoid toxicity.

Bleeding from exposed skeletal muscle can be difficult to cauterize. The use of a topical vasoconstrictor, such as phenylephrine, applied with gauze, may be useful for handling this problem.

When performing Mohs surgery on the ear it is often helpful to balloon up the tissue over the cartilage with the anesthetic solution. This makes it easier to take an additional layer of tissue, if necessary, by limiting the depth of the initial section. Also, if ballooning is achieved, it is an indicator that tumor may not have invaded to cartilage.

Suggested Readings

Adriani J: Labat's regional anesthesia: Techniques and clinical applications. 4th Ed. Warren H Green, St. Louis, 1985

Applegate CN, Fox PT: Neurologic emergencies in internal medicine. p. 473. In Dunagan WC, Ridner ML (eds): Manual of Medical Therapeutics. 26th Ed. Little, Brown, Boston, 1989

Arndt KA, Burton C, Noe JM: Minimizing the pain of local anesthesia. Plast Reconstr Surg 72:676, 1983

Bezzant JL, Stephen RL, Petelenz TJ, Jacobsen SC: Painless cauterization of spider veins with the use of iontophoretic local anesthesia. J Am Acad Dermatol 19:869, 1988

Centers for Disease Control: Guidelines for prevention of transmission of Human Immunodeficiency Virus and Hepatitis B Virus to healthcare and public safety workers. MMWR 38(5–6):1, 1989

Chandler MJ, Grammer LC, Patterson R: Provocative challenge with local anesthesia in patients with a prior history of reaction. J Allergy Clin Immunol 79:883, 1987

Covino BG, Vassallo HG: Local Anesthetics: Mechanisms of Action and Clinical Use. Grune & Stratton, Orlando, FL, 1976.

Defazio CA: Local anesthetics: Action, metabolism, and toxicity. Otolaryngol Clin North Am 14:515, 1981

de Jong RH, Heavner JE: Diazepam prevents local anesthetic seizures. Anesthiology 34:523, 1971

de Jong RH: Local Anesthetics. 2nd Ed. Charles C Thomas, Springfield, IL 1977

Eriksson E: Illustrated handbook in local anesthesia. 2nd Ed. WB Saunders, Philadelphia 1980

Fisher AA: Local anesthetics. p. 220. In Fisher AA (ed): Contact Dermatitis. 3rd Ed. Lea & Febiger, Philadelphia 1986

Fisher DA: Local anesthesia in dermatologic surgery (letter). J Am Acad Dermatol 22:139, 1990

Fisher M: Intradermal testing after anaphylactoid reaction to anaesthetic drugs: Practical aspects of performance and interpretation. Anaesth Intens Care 12:115, 1984

Foster CA, Aston SJ: Propanolol-epinephrine interaction: A potential disaster. Plast Reconstr Surg 72:74, 1983

Grabb WC: A concentration of 1 : 500,000 epinephrine in a local anesthetic solution is sufficient to provide excellent hemostasis (letter). Plast Reconstr Surg 63:834, 1979

Grekin RC, Auletta MJ: Local anesthesia in dermatologic surgery. J Am Acad Dermatol 19:599, 1988

Huff BB (ed): Physician's Desk Reference. Medical Economics, Oradell, NJ, 1987

Juhlin L, Evers H, Borberg F: A lidocaine-prilocaine cream for superficial skin surgery and painful lesions. Acta Derm Venereol (Stockh) 60:544, 1980

Klein JA: Anesthesia for liposuction in dermatologic surgery. J Dermatol Surg Oncol 14:1124, 1988

Lippman M, Rumley W: Medical emergencies. p. 484. In Dunagan WC, Ridner ML (eds): Manual of Medical Therapeutics. Little, Brown, Boston, 1989

Maloney JM III, Lertora JJL, Yarborough J, et al: Plasma concentrations of lidocaine during hair transplantation. J Dermatol Surg Oncol 8:950, 1982

Nattel ST, Rinkenberger RL, Lehrman LL, Zipes DP: Therapeutic blood lidocaine concentrations after local anesthesia for cardiac electrophysiologic studies. N Engl J Med 301:418, 1979

Ritchie JM, Greene NM: Local anesthetics. p. 302. In Gilman AG, Goodman LS, Rall TW, Murad F (eds): The Pharmacological Basis of Therapeutics. 7th Ed. Macmillan, 1985

Serota H: Basic and advanced life cardiac life support. p. 175. In Dunagan WC, Ridner ML (eds): Manual of Medical Therapeutics. Little, Brown, Boston, 1989

Snow JC: Manual of Anesthesia. Little, Brown, Boston, 1982

Index

Page numbers followed by f indicate figures; those followed by t indicate tables.